A LONG TRIAGE
Welcome to My War

By Francis J. Sullivan Jr.

Publisher and Author: Francis J. Sullivan Jr.
                        1 Grace Court
                        Corrales, NM 87048
                        tel: (978) 590-4624
                        email: attyfjs@earthlink.net

Cover and interior
design and editing: Kacia Reilly

Cover Art: James Nelson

Copyright (c) 2025 by Francis J. Sullivan Jr. with original Registration Number TXu-2 118-360. All rights reserved. No reprinting of the text herein without written permission of the copyright holder is allowed. Furthermore, no use of the content herein for any audio, visual or any other reason is allowed without the written permission of the copyright holder. No part of this book may be reproduced or transmitted in any form of electronic or mechanical means including but not limited to photocopying, recording, or by any information storage or retrieval system without permission of the copyholder.

Library of Congress 2020903080

ISBN: 978-1-7340554-0-5

A Long Triage consists of a series of works of creative non-fiction. Although the substance of the story is true and has been experienced by the author, names of people (except his immediate family), places and the sequence of events have been altered in the spirit of poetic license to accommodate the telling of the story in the form presented to the reader.

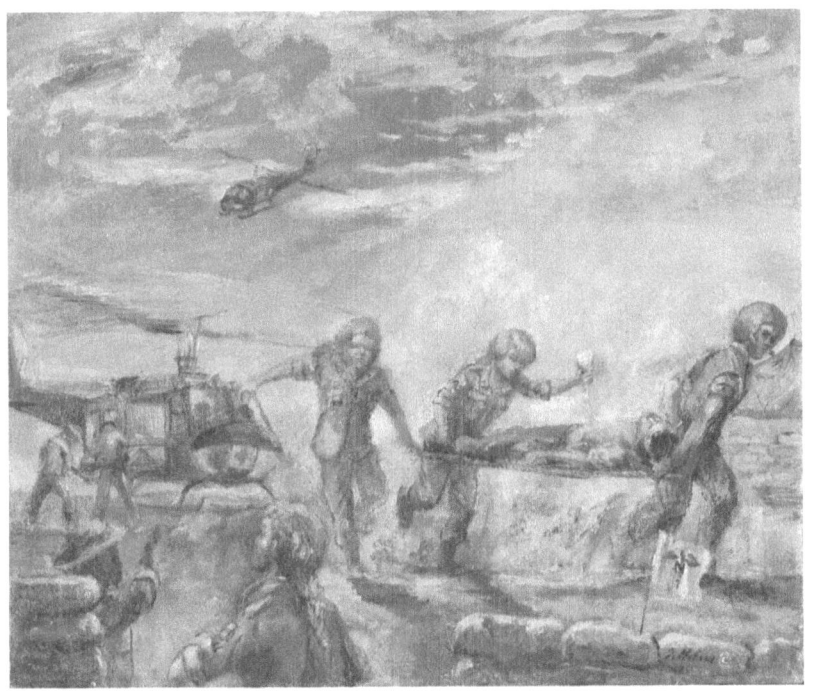

The painting titled "TRIAGE" was created by James Davis Nelson in commemoration of the excellent job done and the sacrifices made by the medical corps of all branches of the American military services during the Vietnam War.

Nelson served in Vietnam from 1967 to 1968 as an infantry rifleman, machine gunner, draftsman and combat artist.

The painting and commemoration inspired the title of this book.

This reproduction is a black and white version of the original.

PROLOGUE

According to military records, 58,222[1] US soldiers died while fighting in America's war in Vietnam. Out of that number, 18,465[2] of those who died were classified as infantry soldiers with a Military Occupational Specialty (MOS) of 11B, infantry riflemen. The other 39,737 Americans who died in the Vietnam War were identified by a variety of other occupational specialties according to their jobs and most of those soldiers supported the infantry during military operations.

In other words, more than 65% of the American deaths during America's war in Vietnam were not 11B infantry rifelman.

In military terminology, the number of soldiers supporting the infantry is T3R, which stands for the tooth-to-tail ratio. It is the number of support personnel (tail soldiers) it takes to supply and support each infantry soldier (tooth soldiers) during combat operations. While both "tooth" and "tail" soldiers may find themselves in combat or other life-threatening situations, infantry soldiers are those whose primary function is to neutralize the enemy. Therefore, the infantry is also referred to as the "Tip of the Spear," while support soldiers are referred to as being at "the Other End." But these terms were not used in the daily language of many infantry soldiers while fighting in Vietnam when they referred to the soldiers supporting them during combat operations.

1. https://www.archives.gov/research/military/vietnam-war/casualty-statistics
2. http://www.uswardogs.org/vietnam-statistics/

RETURNING

The homecoming trail tapered
off into a void

Grave consequence awaited those
forgetting the reasons why

Memories etched upon our souls
Lessons learned

Appreciated and not left behind

Dedicated to Patti, Kacia, Kelsey
and all my family

TABLE OF CONTENTS

Chapter 1 17

Chapter 2 33

Chapter 3 41

Chapter 4 53

Chapter 5 63

Chapter 6 75

Chapter 7 89

Chapter 8 103

Chapter 9 113

Chapter 10 121

Chapter 11 131

Chapter 12 143

Chapter 13 155

Chapter 14 165

A Long Triage

A PATRIOTIC PARADOX

The call of our nation

Causing frustration

Pain to one's heart

From the very start

Soldiers coming home

Deserted and alone

Anger running deep

Penetrating sleep

Lost they are

Emotional scar

Vietnam being lost

Such a wasteful cost

A Long Triage

CHAPTER ONE

SEPTEMBER 1968 – OCTOBER 1969:

They called us rear echelon motherfuckers, even when they knew our names. REMFs for short. Not all of them, but enough of them to piss me off. They were no different than the schoolyard bullies I fought against when I was a kid.

When they harassed me, and tried to intimidate me, I wanted to let them die or kill them myself. But that wasn't going to be good for any of us. In reality, whether we wanted to admit it or not, we depended on each other to stay alive.

They were grunts, infantry soldiers fighting in the worst conditions of combat. We were the troops providing them with the support they needed for their missions.

But we weren't one of them. So, they treated us like shit.

They were jealous of us because we had more creature comforts at our bases of operation than they had out in the bush: beds, showers, and hot food just to name a few. And their lives were often in more obvious danger than ours. But I refused to accept their derisive attitude towards us. We were all soldiers serving our country during America's war in Vietnam. We were supposed to be "Brothers in Arms" fighting for a common cause in support of our Nation.

****

I've tried to put my tour of duty in Vietnam behind me and manage my emotions, but the memories haven't disappeared. They still haunt me. Regularly. And too often they flood my mind with daydreams, nightmares, and flashbacks of my own close calls with death and impact my daily life in very real and very destructive ways.

I survived my tour of duty in Vietnam and came home physically in one piece. I was lucky, and I'm grateful. But even now, more than fifty years later, unexpected events trigger memories that rekindle my fear of injury or death, stoke the resentment I have for that period in my life and cause me to have outbursts and out-of-body experiences.

At first, I hear fluttering in my ears. Then I hear whistling followed by flashes of light that blind me. Sometimes I panic and dive to the ground. I'm frightened, and I wait for the sounds of the explosions I'm sure will follow. My heart pounds rapidly, blood rushes to my head in pulsating aching throbs, and my mind spins like a child's toy top. I'm back in Vietnam, cramped into the fetal position, my eyes piercing the sky waiting to die.

Other times, I stay somewhat grounded, but I lose focus. I perceive any little unexpected event as life threatening. My fight-or-flight response kicks in. I lose control. I can't tell friend from foe. My temper flares up, and I aggressively defend myself from the people around me: my face turns red; my voice becomes crackly and loud, and the people I'm with move away from me to avoid the confrontation.

My doctors have told me that I suffer from Post-Traumatic Stress Disorder (PTSD). And they call these episodes "startled reactions" triggered by the unexpected events.

Usually after a short time, my heart slows down, my mind clears, the pulsating throbs fade away, and life resumes a somewhat normal course. But this most recent episode has been the worst of them all and seems to be never-ending.

****

JANUARY 17, 2014:

The last thing I remember before waking up in a hospital bed surrounded by a team of doctors was eating lunch at a restaurant with a group of my fellow court appointed attorneys. My cell phone vibrated in my shirt pocket. So, I excused myself from the table, left the restaurant, sat in my car, and answered the call.

It was Annie, one of the probation officers I worked with on a regular basis. I was used to the way she always seemed to act with superiority over court appointed attorneys. But this time her attitude was unacceptable.

"Attorney Sullivan," She said. "I wish you hadn't gone to lunch. It's Friday and I have the afternoon off."

"Annie, I went to lunch at the close of morning session, like everybody else."

"Well I'm going to ask the judge to send your client back to jail before I leave. I've got plans for the rest of the day and I can't wait for you to get back here. I'll get someone else to cover the case."

"I can be there in half an hour."

"Don't bother rushing back to court for this case. It will be done before you get here."

I couldn't believe what I was hearing. An image of her pale freckled face with the map of Ireland written all over it surrounded by her fiery red hair flashed in front of me. It was the grunts versus the REMFs all over again.

"Bullshit," I screamed into the phone. "You're violating my client's constitutional right to counsel," I shouted at the top of my lungs.

"Not really, he'll have an attorney."

"But he has a right to his own attorney. And that's me."

"Take it up with the judge, when you get here."

When she said that, I could taste the anger burning my throat. The fluttering and whistling of rockets and mortars punctured my ears, a pain exploded in my head like a bomb and traveled through my blood vessels and nerves to my stomach. I became nauseous, began vomiting profusely, and everything turned black.

****

I woke up a couple days later lying in the hospital bed.

Bright fluorescent ceiling lights blurred my vision. And the noise in the room was earsplitting. But I could hear the doctors talking to my wife, Patti and my daughter Kacia.

"Mrs. Sullivan, when he arrived by ambulance his brain was hemorrhaging. So, we performed an emergency craniotomy and evacuated an actively bleeding subdural hematoma. Do you know how he hit his head?"

"As far as I know he didn't hit his head. This whole thing came out of nowhere."

"Why do you say that?"

"When his friends called and told me he was being brought to the hospital, they said he had been eating lunch with them and just stepped outside to answer a phone call. One of his friends went to see why he was taking so long and found him unconscious sitting behind the wheel of his car. So, he called 911."

"It's a good thing he did. He saved his life. Spontaneous Subdural Hematomas can be fatal."

"Will he recover?"

"We'll have to wait and see. He had an adverse reaction to the anesthesia. As the anesthesia wore off, he was in a state of delirium screaming incoherently about REMFs and grunts, incoming rockets and mortars, and gooks coming through the wire."

"Under those conditions I'm not surprised. He does that when he wakes up from nightmares about Vietnam."

"How long has that been going on?"

"As long as I've known him. He was diagnosed with PTSD about twenty years ago, went through a psychotic break and tried to commit suicide. Then about ten years later he had a similar episode when he had open-heart surgery."

****

All kinds of medications were prescribed for me to take for a variety of reasons. But the one that concerned me the most was Dilantin. Evidently seizures could be a possible side effect as a result of my brain surgery.

A psychiatrist was added to my team of caregivers. My rehabilitation and recovery included physical therapy, occupational therapy, and speech therapy for the brain injury and symptoms of stroke. And psychotherapy was added to help me with my PTSD.

My goal became threefold. Not only would I need to

overcome my physical symptoms, I needed to get the reality of my experiences during the war into focus and purge myself of some deep-seated anger, which the doctors said was most likely not only related to my experiences in the war but related to my life experiences before Vietnam and after coming home from Vietnam.

****

They kept me in the hospital for a few more weeks. But the hospital was not properly equipped to handle patients with delirium. Not all of the staff had been properly trained to accommodate a patient requiring sensory deprivation therapy. The environment surrounding me was too busy and too noisy. I felt like I was stuck in a subway station with no idea where to go.

When the nurses and other staff members came into my room, they would turn on the lights and leave the door open. I could hear the conversations of people in the hallway clear down to the nurse's station that was at the end of a long hollow tunnel. People came in and out of my room all day and night waking me up to check my vital signs and would forget to close the door and turn off the bright ceiling lights as they left.

Because I was under doctor's orders not to get out of bed without assistance, I'd press the call button for someone to come back and turn off the lights and close the door. But by the time someone came back to my room it would be time for more invasive procedures to my body. And the irritating cycle would start all over again.

So, I went without sleep for several days at a time, remained in an agitated state and continually engaged in arguments with the staff. Throughout that time, all I could think about was getting out of there.

After several more days of enduring this egregious and unhealthy environment, a friendly doctor with a soothing voice came into my room and introduced himself as Doctor Alok Ransing.

His appearance caught me off guard. I went into a kind of mental tailspin. I thought I was looking at some hippie from back in the 1960s. He was a handsome guy, about six feet tall, and thin. He was probably in his early thirties. He had a noticeably round face, a dark complexion that was almost mahogany in color, and the large, round eyes I've always associated with people from India.

The hippy look came from his kurta, a traditional shirt worn by people in his eastern culture. I remember seeing the followers of the Hare Krishna movement and the radical hippies wearing clothes like his during the anti-war protests that were occurring all around America back in those days.

I sat there like a zombie staring at him with a blank look on my face thinking about how the protesters had sabotaged my return home from the war. I don't know how long he waited for me to respond, but when I came to my senses he was no longer in my room.

****

While I was eating breakfast in bed the next day, there was someone knocking on the door to my room.

"Good morning Mr. Sullivan. It's Doctor Ransing. We met yesterday. I'm the psychiatrist that has been assigned to be in charge of your treatment team. May I come in?"

"Yes of course. Nice to meet you Doctor Ransing. Good morning to you too. Sorry about blanking out yesterday."

"How do you feel this morning?"

"Disoriented."

"That's understandable, considering the circumstances."

"What do you mean?"

"Mr. Sullivan, you just survived brain surgery, which is a serious operation for anybody to undergo. And seeing that you had an adverse reaction to the anesthesia and emerged from it in a state of delirium with the symptoms of a stroke I was not surprised by your catatonic state yesterday."

"So, you don't think I'm crazy?"

"No, I don't think you're crazy. But after reading your medical and psychiatric reports I see other complications that we will need to deal with during your recovery that concern me."

"Well I have concerns too doctor. But most of my concerns right now have to do with the lack of respect most of the staff has for my condition."

"What do you mean, Mr. Sullivan?"

I gave him a detailed explanation of the irritating conditions that had been going on up to that point in time.

"I apologize for the problem. I will definitely speak to the nursing supervisor."

"Thank you for understanding, Doctor."

"You're welcome. This won't resolve all of my other

concerns though."

"What are your other concerns?"

"Well, on the surface you appear to be one of the lucky Vietnam veterans because you came home in one piece and adjusted fairly well to civilian life."

"I don't know if I can agree with that."

"I'm just referring to the basic facts. You got married, stayed employed, raised a family, and graduated from college and law school."

"Yes Doctor, that's true. But I've had to work hard at keeping myself under control while doing those things. And I was not always successful."

"Yes, I can see that from reading your records and talking with your family."

"What'd they say?"

"They've told me that for the first twenty years after you returned home and managed to accomplish those things, you regularly lashed out in anger at the people around you while self-medicating with alcohol and drugs. You smashed up several motor vehicles, had a psychotic break, and tried to kill yourself."

"Yes, that's true as well. But back then I was on a strange cocktail of medications that made everything worse, and I didn't want to hurt other people. So, I took it out on myself."

"Well, we'd like to keep that from happening again."

"So would I. How do we do that?"

"Your treatment team has developed a partial discharge plan to get you home."

"That's great to hear."

"We are scheduling you for speech therapy, physical therapy, and occupational therapy for your medical conditions on a daily basis in your home for several months. And we are recommending Narrative Therapy for your PTSD."

"What does that actually mean, Narrative Therapy? I've been through about every type of therapy program there is for PTSD."

"Yes, I know you have. But now you will also be dealing with the symptoms of a traumatic brain injury."

"So, how is this going to be any different than those other therapeutic programs?"

Doctor Ransing spent quite a bit of time explaining that the other programs were structured around the person being a problem. But in Narrative Therapy the patient is not seen as the problem, the events in the patient's life that trigger the psychotic episodes are seen as the problems.

He recommended that I write a narrative about my memories of serving in Vietnam. He assured me that the experience would be therapeutic because it would let me see the events that happened there as separate from me. As a result, he said, I would develop a better understanding of the problems I was having in the past. And he said that with help from my treatment team, I could learn to control my reactions to events that may startle me in the future.

He asked me to continue writing at home after I was discharged from the hospital and that when I was finished to schedule an appointment at his out-patient mental health clinic and bring my written work with me when I came for my first appointment.

****

A week later I was finally discharged from the hospital, although I continued to exhibit the symptoms of stroke. I still couldn't see clearly or identify whole objects. For instance, I would eat half the food on my plate because I couldn't see the other half. Then either Patti or Kacia or my son Kelsey would spin the plate and I'd see the rest of the food and continue eating. Sometimes I had trouble speaking so we had to communicate with hand signals and note pads.

To make matters worse, I couldn't keep my balance or walk without assistance. Fortunately, we lived in a garden-level apartment with no stairs at the front entrance. So, I was able to get inside without much trouble. But once I was inside the apartment, Patti or one of the kids needed to help me manage my daily activities: showering, shaving, dressing, and being reminded of the order in which the activities were to be done.

Kacia had flown out from California where she lived and worked as a graphic designer. She helped Patti get me home and settled in. But she had to get back to work. Before she left, Kelsey came down from Maine, where he lived and worked as a bird biologist.

I was grateful that both our children had committed themselves to alternating as caregivers alongside Patti until we could manage on our own. And the interactions we had through this ordeal gave me a sense of pride and appreciation beyond description. Our children had grown up to be responsible and caring successful adults. As a parent, I couldn't ask for more.

The hospital had arranged for the outpatient team to provide me with the services I needed in our home until

I could commute to the outpatient mental health clinic. Each day of the work week, a different therapist came to our home and worked with me for a couple hours doing different activities: balancing exercises, writing, drawing, speaking with clarity, and moving my eyes in circles and reverse circles to help eliminate the visual disturbances. And a nurse arrived once a week to take blood samples for the lab and check my vital signs.

The in-home routine went on for several months. During that time, I felt like a child. The stroke like symptoms kept reoccurring on a daily basis. And I had to keep learning how to walk, talk, and write all over again. But I took Doctor Ransing's advice, instead of keeping my anger bottled up inside I put my energy into gaining my skills back and writing my therapeutic narrative.

CHAPTER TWO

MARCH 11, 1968:

My problems with the Army started before I was sent to Vietnam. I had already signed papers to join the Navy. My friend Matt had joined with me on what was known at the time as the buddy system. It meant we would be in basic training together. But he was still in his draft deferred educational program, and I had flunked out of college and lost my student deferment. So, you could say that I caused my own problem with the Army.

We passed our mental and physical examinations, and initially we had been put on a one-hundred and twenty-day delay status to allow us to finish out the school year. Matt and I had been scheduled to be sworn into the Navy in June. In the meantime, I received a letter from my local draft board ordering me to report to the

Boston Army Base for a pre-induction physical examination.

When I arrived, a uniformed recruiter, standing tall, ridged, and wearing a big smirk across his face greeted me.

"Mr. Sullivan," he said. "Someone has to take the place of the conscientious objector from your hometown that refused to be drafted. And you are next on the list."

This news took me by surprise. I was really bummed out. I had planned to follow in my father's footsteps. He had joined the Navy and served in the South Pacific during world War II. And his colorful stories of going around the world and crossing the equator had intrigued me when I was a child.

"But I've already joined the Navy," I protested.

"Tough shit," he said. "Don't be such a pussy. There's nothing I can do about it. We have quotas that need to be filled, bodies to send to Vietnam. Just get in line with the rest of these poor bastards."

It was the beginning of a long and uncomfortable day. I got in line with hundreds of kids my age. We were directed through a series of stations which seemed designed to treat us like cattle in a herd of dumb animals.

Welcome to My War

The bully behavior of basic training had already started, and we hadn't even been sworn into the Army yet.

"Move along in single file," was the constant shout that was repeated over and over again as the herd moved through the processing stations.

"Strip to your shorts but leave your socks on. Put the rest of your personal shit in the plastic bags that PFC Garcia hands you on your way to station two," was the command at station one. At station two we were given a bunch of shots with a variety of needles vaccinating us for all kinds of diseases. But nobody told us what they were.

All day long it went on like that: doctors and nurses checking our vital signs: blood pressure, blood samples, heart rate, temperature, eyes and ears checked. And for most people the bend over spread your cheeks and cough exam was the worst of them all. But for me the worst part was the last station.

For a short time, I felt relieved that the ordeal was about to end. And I'd be going home for supper. But at the last station, the line was broken into two directions. Line A was for pre-induction. Line B was for induction. I reached the entrance to the last station and heard the shouts of the sergeants in charge.

"Put your fucking clothes back on and get into the line

that applies to your sorry ass. And hand your paperwork to the men at the desks."

As I was getting dressed, I kept thinking about getting home for supper and figuring out a way to move up my date to be sworn into the Navy, even if that meant starting my basic training without Matt. But that moment was short lived.

After I finished putting my clothes back on, I waited in line A for my turn to hand the man at the desk what I thought were my pre-induction papers. Much to my amazement when I passed my papers to him, he laughed and raised his voice. Everyone must have heard what he said.

"Sullivan, Francis J, we've been waiting for you. Big surprise sailor boy you're in the Army now."

I looked all around. It seemed like everyone was staring at me. It was embarrassing. I was nervous but couldn't let it show. So, I gave the man a big salute, like it was all a big joke.

He reached under his desk and pulled out a box labeled "US Navy" in bright blue letters on the cover. He took some papers out of the box: put them down on his desk. I was shocked when I saw that they were my Navy papers. He stamped them with big red letters that said "PRE-INDUCTION."

It's been more than fifty years since that day, and I still get angry when I think of that moment. I can even picture the little brown cardboard box with the Navy's emblem: a gold rope circling the insignia, the eagle defending a ship, and my name embossed over the middle of it all, identifying me as a new recruit for the Navy.

The irony of the situation still astonishes me when I think about it. I took the place of one of my friends from back home. But he had the balls to challenge the government. He refused to be drafted because he claimed that America's presence in the war in Vietnam was not justified.

I remember the harassment and intimidation that people in my hometown tormented him and his family with when his case made the news on the front page of the local papers and appeared on local television channels. But the government backed off and did nothing to him. And all I wanted to do was join the Navy instead of the Army.

"Sullivan, get your ass over to Line B for induction and hand your pre-induction paperwork to the man at the desk, before I give you a boot in the ass."

I moved over to line B and for the second time that day I handed my papers to a man at a desk. He took my Navy papers from my left hand and put them down on his desk. Then he took the papers I had accumulated during the day from my right hand and stamped them "INDUCTION."

"Welcome to the Army Mr. Draftee Sullivan the Sailor Man. Follow that line to your right and get on one of the busses outside."

"But this was only supposed to be my day for pre-induction. I've already joined the Navy. My family thinks I'll be home for supper."

"That's too bad. You're in the Army now. Complaining won't get you anywhere. Get on one of the busses or we'll have you arrested, and you can complain to a judge."

My heart sank so deep I was afraid I was going to cry in front of a few hundred guys who were as unhappy about getting drafted as I was. So, I took it all on the chin—maned-up as the saying goes—and moved along with the rest of the line.

There were four busses sitting outside in the parking lot. I got on bus number three. When all the busses were full, they left Boston and headed South on Interstate 95. After an hour or so of me pleading with the bus driver about my poor family expecting me home for supper, I finally convinced him to make a stop at a Howard Johnson restaurant and let me call home and tell my family what had happened. But when the bus was loaded up again and the driver took a head count, he came over to me with an angry look on his face.

"Hey buddy I'm probably going to lose my job on account of you."

"What did I do?"

"I never should have listened to you. I just took a head count and we're missing two people."

"Sorry about that. But my mom really appreciated knowing why I hadn't showed up for supper."

"That's great, but it doesn't help me."

Buses one, two, and three pulled into Fort Dix New Jersey for Army basic training. Bus four kept going South on Route 95. The bus driver started laughing loud enough for all of us new recruits to hear him. "You guys think you've got it bad. Bus four is headed for Parris Island. Those poor bastards will be Marines, whether they want to or not."

****

Boot camp was actually fun for me. I was in good physical condition from playing sports throughout my childhood and school years. After boot camp, I attended signal school at Fort Gordon Georgia. I had already been trained as an electrician by my father from the time I was twelve years old so, studying circuitry was easy for me.

All through military training everyone is expected to put up with the bully behavior of the drill sergeants and instructors. I continually placed myself in the middle of the crowd every chance I had. That strategy helped me avoid being singled out to be harassed and intimidated by the instructors.

My only real problem during my training came when I was sent home on leave to attend a family funeral. Some of the guys I was training with became jealous. They were upset because I had been doing so well with my training the instructors didn't require me to make up the time or the work I missed.

I refused to accept their attempts at intimidation and harassment. And upon graduation, I expected respect to be shown to each other as fellow soldiers. As it turns out, I was quite naive to have had such an unrealistic expectation.

CHAPTER THREE

SEPTEMBER 1968:

Along with more than two hundred of my fellow American soldiers I boarded a commercial airliner in Oakland, California. The plane had been contracted by the United States government to fly replacement troops into the war zone. Some of us had been drafted. Some of us had volunteered. But we had all been ordered to serve in Vietnam.

The mood was an odd blend of calm and anxiety. Some soldiers looked like stoic marble portraits prepared for anything that may come their way. Others seemed carefree: laughing, joking, playing card games, and teasing each other like brothers. A few appeared ready to burst into tears. I think I was one of the stoic one's but inside, I was simply afraid of what the next year of my life would be like, and I hoped that I could handle myself like a man and make my family proud of me. But most of all I wondered how many of us would be alive and in one piece at the end of the year. We flew to Hawaii, changed flight crews, made a stop in Japan to refuel, and then flew on to Vietnam.

As the plane approached the military base in Ben Hoa, Vietnam, I could see red and yellow flames flickering against the dark-night sky surrounding the airfield. After the plane landed, we stepped off the plane and entered a damp, murky world that reeked of death like the putrid mist of composting rotten vegetation. It was alarming but not unexpected. After all, by the time we left California we had been trained and prepared for combat. But morning came with a shock that military training hadn't prepared me for.

After breakfast, I was the last man standing in the company formation surrounded by a field of sand with the beautiful clear-blue South China Sea in the background. The sergeant of the guard handed me an M14 rifle, led me into an olive-drab Army tent filled with an eerie translucent smoke. He sat me down in front of an American GI perched upon a wooden bench and shackled to an ammunition can.

Many years have passed since then. So, I'm not exactly sure of everything that happened that day. But in my recurring nightmare the sergeant says, "Private Sullivan, this is Billy. Keep your eyes on him. Last night the dumb shit killed one of my best men over a stupid poker game."

"Not true," says Billy. "It was self-defense. Sully, just wait and see. You'll learn lots of strange things here in the Nam."

As the sergeant turns to leave, he says, "Sullivan stay with him till the MPs come and get him. Shoot him if he tries to get away."

My knees started to shake, perspiration covered my forehead, and I was freaked out wondering if this was really happening. But I said, "Yes, Sergeant."

Sitting there on either end of the bench, Billy and I must have looked like book ends: five-feet-8 inches in height, 160 pounds, blackish brown hair, and dressed in jungle fatigues. He could have been any one of a thousand guys who were drafted with me at 19 years of age that spring.

Throughout the day, I escorted Billy to the mess hall, the piss tubes, and the shit house. All three were in separate locations around the base. He carried the ammo can shackled to his wrists. And I trailed behind him: my weapon locked and loaded, ready for action with sweat soaking through my uniform, and a flushing fluid heat pulsating through every blood vessel in my body.

Before the day was over, he practically told me his whole life story. The similarities between us were striking: we were about the same age, from small-town America, and raised in large families by second-generation Welsh/Irish, Roman Catholic parents. Our parents were members of Tom Brokaw's Greatest Generation: church going, hard-working, World War II veterans.

When we got our draft notices, we had no real choice. We had to go, or risk being called cowards and disowned by our families and communities.

Billy had been called after graduating from high school. I made it through a partial year of college before flunking out and losing my student deferment.

****

Billy told me he had been in-country for almost a year and was preparing to go home when the shooting incident occurred. Then he warned me of the difficult choices I would need to make in order to survive my tour of duty in Vietnam. His cautions addressed both the enemy and our own people:

>Whether to trust or not trust somebody,

>Whether to fall asleep or stay awake on guard duty,

Whether to hang out with the juicers or the pot heads,

Whether to volunteer for patrols and ambushes or keep a low profile,

Whether to kill someone or let them live.

His claim of self-defense sounded inconceivable to me at the time. I never expected the animosity between groups of soldiers in a combat zone to be so juvenile and result in such serious consequences. But it didn't take long for me to believe his story might be true.

Billy said, "A group of infantry soldiers came in from the bush to use our company area for a stand-down."

"What's that?" I asked.

"Rest and relaxation. Sometimes it's called in-country R&R. Grunts are out in the boonies most of the time: no showers, sleeping on the ground, eating c-rations. So, they come back here and do all their horsing around, having fun, drinking, pot smoking…and whatever."

"And that's a problem?"

"It wasn't, until they started bragging about being better soldiers than me and my friends. The grunts were deliberately speaking loud enough for us to overhear them during their card game. They were putting us down and bragging about themselves."

As I listened to Billy's story, it was obvious that he and his friends took the insults personally as harassment and intimidation, and a lot of tension built up between the two groups. Then Billy raised his voice.

"Those grunts told us we were lucky to be back in the rear with the gear and not out in the bush where the real war was going on. The bastards called us REMFs."

I didn't know what to believe. But it was clear that Billy's group reacted defensively and competitively. It sounded like they tried to out talk the grunts, contending that just because their jobs were not to go out in the bush and kill the enemy, their positions were dangerous, and their lives were in jeopardy, too.

Neither Billy nor I were gung-ho glory hounds seeking adventure with some kind of morbid interest in killing, like some of the guys we met in the service. We just wanted to do the right thing for our country; whatever that was supposed to be. Answer the call of duty, even if it scared the hell out of you and you didn't understand the big picture? We had been raised to believe that the morality of war was the responsibility of our fearless leaders. So, follow orders, suck it up, and be a man.

Billy relaxed and went on with his story.

"It's our job to support the infantry, so we're stuck in bunkers relaying radio signals, pulling guard duty, and getting shot at day and night. We live through shit storms inside the wire, and gooks are always trying to sneak through the wire to get into the base to cut our throats, plant their explosives, and get out without being seen. Yeah, out in the bush the grunts have it bad: humping through the boonies, setting ambushes, and going on search and destroy missions. But what do they know about our jobs? We could be killed at any time, day or night."

"What are shit storms?" I asked.

"It's what we call the rocket and mortar attacks when the whole area lights up with explosions coming from some place out of the sky."

After I was in country for a short time, I found out the hard way the reasons Billy and his buddies felt the way they did. As support troops, we were always stuck inside the perimeter like sitting ducks with no means of defending ourselves from an enemy we couldn't see. Eventually, I felt the same aggravation and frustration Billy's group experienced, and the emotional toll it took on them ... and finally took on me. But in that moment, I still didn't know what to think.

During my own tour of duty, not only did I experience the same conditions as Billy and the guys around him, but also, I resented the irony. We were support troops performing a variety of tasks necessary for the infantry to be successful, but we were trapped. Trapped behind the wire and exposed to danger just like those sitting ducks.

Our support was required for all kinds of things, including communication, transportation, medical aid, air support, and artillery. The paradox being that not only did the success of the infantry soldiers' missions depend on us, the number of casualties would increase without our support—the support provided by the very same soldiers the grunts were harassing and intimidating with their contempt.

But I didn't know any of that at the time. Billy was the first to clue me in. He was heated again.

"At least the grunts can defend themselves. They can even run away from the in-coming fire if they want, and believe me, some do. But support troops can't run away. We're stuck inside the wire doing our jobs in the middle of these shit storms. And the reality is, we're the targets of the incoming fire."

I'll never forget the look of anger on Billy's face as he spoke. He appeared to be ready to explode into a rage. But after several minutes, he calmed down again and continued with the story of what really happened that fatal night.

"Two other guys were in the bunker with me the night of the shooting. At my court-martial, they can testify that not only was there a poker game the night before the shooting, the grunts were making other bets among themselves."

"What were they betting on?" I asked.

"My friends overheard them betting that during the night they could sneak into our bunkers along the perimeter, catch us off guard, and prove that they were better soldiers than us—that REMFs weren't real warriors."

Billy swore the card game and the grunts badmouthing the support troops had nothing to do with the shooting.

He said, "The evidence at my court-martial will prove the grunts tried to go through with their stupid game of sneaking into our bunker. Only problem was, they failed to give the password when I challenged them while they were crawling around outside of our bunker in the dark."

"What do you mean?" I asked.

"The grunts tried to worm their way through an area where we had tied strings of tin cans together. We left some in the dirt and bundled some around the entrance to our bunker for extra precaution. In the middle of the night, I heard the cans rattle and screamed, 'Charlotte.' They should have replied, 'Greensborough.' But nobody responded. So, I started shooting because I thought the enemy was breaching our perimeter."

"Then it was their fault,"

"Yes, but it doesn't matter. They'll charge me with murder anyway."

Our trip around the airbase revealed a common attitude from the troops. Evidently, the story of the shooting had circulated among the men. As we walked from place to place, I heard several soldiers call out: "Shoot the bastard, shoot the bastard." Some of them harassed me for being a replacement troop new to Vietnam, a "cherry" according to them, and a REMF because I wouldn't shoot Billy.

As far as I'm concerned, Billy and the guy he killed were tragic victims of the government's poor training of young men for war.

Looking back, I guess it's not surprising. In addition to the actual physical training and weapons training to prepare us for battle, the government used brainwashing strategies during our training to manipulate our minds to make us become killers: marching, singing, and chanting:

> I want to be an airborne ranger.
>
> I want to live a life of danger.
>
> I want to go to Vietnam.
>
> I want to kill the Viet Cong.
>
> Sound off. . .One two.
>
> Sound off. . .Three four.
>
> I want to go and fight in the war.
>
> I want to even the score
>
> kill . . . kill . . . kill
>
> just for the thrill . . . thrill . . . thrill.
>
> On your left . . . left . . . left . . . right . . . left.
>
> 1-2-3-4, off we go to fight the war.

Although Billy and I exchanged addresses with the intention to keep in touch with each other, I was relieved when the MPs came and took him off my hands. I returned the M14 to the sergeant of the guard, went back to the barracks, laid down on my bunk and tossed and turned throughout a sleepless night.

CHAPTER FOUR

After roll call the next day, a group of screaming sergeants rounded up all the cherries, corralled us together, herded us into a cattle car, delivered us to a stockyard serving as an airstrip, and packed us like sardines into a C-130 transport plane. We were beasts headed to the slaughterhouse. The atmosphere was rank with the body odor of a high-school locker room. Through the flames of blasting rockets and mortars, we rose into the sky above the razor-sharp metal wire surrounding the perimeter of the enclave and headed north.

Passenger accommodations in those "garbage scows of the air" were sparse. There were no seats. We sat on bare metal skids and cargo pallets normally used for shipping supplies like trucks, tanks, and explosives. A spindle-shaped, metal-clad tunnel of a fuselage surrounded us, and a crosshatched geodesic superstructure of welded struts and tubing supported the tunnel. It was a metal fishing net and we were the catch of the day.

With our fully packed duffel bags for cushions and canvas tie-down straps for safety belts, we were prepared for a combat landing. With no windows or lighting within the confines of the dark, cavernous cargo compartment, I became hypnotized by the incessant drone of the engines and rhythmic banging and rattling of every rivet, nut, and bolt holding the aircraft together and drifted into a trance.

My daydream had me flying into fire all over again, reliving the smell of the foul odor of death from the first landing. I was convinced it was a menacing prelude to the inevitable explosions I was sure would blow us all away.

In my imagination, I hovered above the plane with an image of Billy in my brain. He was in his bunker screaming, "Charlotte," and firing his rifle into the night. With my mind floating somewhere in the distance, I could see the plane landing safely in Chu Lai.

****

Back then, Chu Lai was a United States Marine airfield with operational centers for several Army infantry units supported by the Navy, the Air Force, and the Coast Guard. The whole complex sat along the coast of the South China Sea, 580 miles south of Hanoi and 480 miles north of what was still Saigon, the capital of South Vietnam during the war when it was an independent nation. After the war, Chu Lai became a major seaport with an international airport and is now an important part of our global economy, while Hanoi is now the capital of Vietnam and Saigon, merging with the surrounding province, is now Ho Chi Minh City.

If you were to look at a map of Vietnam showing the boundaries in place during the 1960s and 1970s, south of Hanoi and far to the north of Saigon you would find a boundary labeled demilitarized zone, or DMZ. Theoretically, the line represented neutrality and acted as a buffer zone between the nations engaged in the conflict. But, in reality, the area was a highly contested and dangerous place.

Below the DMZ, the United States military and political powers established four theaters of operation in South Vietnam. These areas were the designated regions within South Vietnam for tactical operations by two or more military divisions under the command of a general. They were identified in sections titled I CORP in the north, and continuing in a southerly direction as II CORP, III CORP, and IV CORP respectively. Chu Lai was in the I CORP theater of operations, with Da Nang and Hue City to the north and Khe San to the west.

****

After all the cherries were off the plane, we marched in formation from the airstrip to the Chu Lai Replacement Center, a dreary place. It looked like a city of tents pitched upon wooden platforms, with plank catwalks connecting the entire site. The maze was constructed over a seamless blanket of sand bordered by the ocean.

Below the catwalks were trenches half full of a murky liquid comprised of red clay and water mixed with sand. Rats as big as cats occupied the trenches frantically looking for scraps of food. We were there to replace soldiers who had been wounded, killed in action, or going home at the end of their tours. Once again, we went through long lines for central processing, medical evaluation, paperwork, and to be assigned a bunk for the night.

"Repple Depple," someone called out when the replacement center staff finished assigning us to our bunks, showed us where the bathroom facilities were located and left us alone.

"What's Repple Depple?" I asked.

The guy that said it responded, "It's what they called replacement centers during WWII. At least that's what my uncle told me before I left for Vietnam. He said back then the Army called these places replacement depots because they were usually at a train station. And he warned me about the guys who staff them."

"What did he warn you about?"

"Their attitude."

"What about it?"

"These guys have no espirit de corps," he said. "Like us fighting men, no pride in their work. They just herd us like cattle and treat us like baggage that needs to be moved from place to place. You know, like the conductors at a train station back home."

"They're just doing their job." I said.

"They're just REMFs and will never see action." He snapped back at me. "They act like they've had a tough tour of duty even though they spend all their time back here in the rear with the gear."

In light of my experience guarding Billy, I was offended by what this guy had just said. He was as much of a cherry as me and had no idea what he was talking about. So, I ignored him, held my tongue, and was glad when he finally fell asleep and I could get some rest.

In the morning after breakfast, all the new guys had to

get into military formation for an assignment to a work detail while we waited for our permanent duty assignments. I was ordered to load up into a two-and-a-half-ton, canvas-covered utility truck called a deuce and a half, with a group of replacement troops going to the beach to fill sandbags for building and reinforcing the bunkers along the outer perimeter of the base.

As the truck rumbled towards the beach over a mucky path through the sand, we heard the rat-tat-tat of rifle fire close by. The tall, weather-beaten gung-ho infantry sergeant that was in charge of the detail screamed, "Get used to that sound and don't worry about it unless our perimeter gets overrun. Meanwhile, us infantry soldiers will protect you FNGs."

"What's an FNG?" I asked the guy next to me.

"Fucking New Guys," he whispered.

We arrived at the remains of an old French villa half buried in the sand. The window openings and doors were empty cavities. The walls were pock marked from rifle fire and partially blown out by rockets and mortars. It was like a movie set, created to film some long-lost ancient ruins.

"Take a good look at what's left of the French," said the sergeant.

The atmosphere around us was a virtual steam bath: oppressive with heat, humidity, and insects. We shoveled sand into bags for several hours with the sun beating down on us. After the truck was finally loaded, we were allowed to swim and cool off.

Like most enlisted men, we took full advantage of the freedom. Not only did we swim, we tied about 100 feet of rope to the back of the duz'n half and towed each other on a piece of wood behind the truck along the tide line, like we were water skiing behind a speedboat.

When it was my turn, I swung out over the tops of the breaking waves and out of voice range from the crew. A helicopter flew overhead, and I could hear the whop-whop-whop of the rotating blades and feel the whirlwind they created. It was a spooky feeling and made me feel unsettled. Next thing I knew, a man falls out from the side door of the helicopter and lands pretty close to me. It scared the shit out of me. In a panic, I dove off the slab of wood.

I started swimming towards him, thinking I could help him. As I got closer, I could see that he was already dead. Before I could gather my wits together, the frothing white water of the breaking waves swallowed the corpse and washed it away. I swam to shore and reported the incident to the sergeant in charge.

Ignoring my terrified voice, with a condescending

smirk across his face, he said, "It was probably just military intelligence officers conducting interrogations on the way back from a fire fight. Forget about it, and don't be such a REMF."

But I couldn't forget what had happened. At suppertime, I decided to seek some comfort by visiting my cousin Michael who happened to be stationed in Chu Lai. While in basic training I had received a letter from home, my mom had written about him and where he was stationed.

He worked as an interpreter with the Military Intelligence Detachment in Chu Lai and was responsible for prisoner interrogations. Although he wasn't a close relative, I thought a family member could help me wrap my head around my experience at the beach.

Chu Lai was a large sprawling military compound with airstrips and helicopter pads practically everywhere I looked. I flagged down an MP driving by in a jeep and told him where I wanted to go.

"I'm headed that way now. Hop in." He said.

"Great, thanks a lot."

I climbed aboard his jeep. When we arrived, I thought I was looking at a kennel. Cages were spread around the marsh. But instead of dogs there were people inside.

I hadn't seen Michael since we were kids, but I still recognized him. He had always looked like the typical Welshman: dark hair, dark eyes, tough build, but taller than the rest of the family. And there he was, right in front of me. I'd have recognized him anywhere.

After we greeted each other, I confided in him, describing the details of my experience at the beach. His response to my concern was disheartening.

"You'll get used to shit like that here in the Nam. It's okay to be a cherry, but don't be a REMF. We were interrogating some Viet Cong we captured during the night. The one you saw us throw out of the chopper wouldn't talk. But you better believe—the next one did."

His attitude upset me even more, but I sucked it up like the man I was supposed to be.

"Yeah, I can handle it, but I wanted to make sure I had the story straight in my mind."

"I know what you mean," he said. "People that haven't been here just don't believe you when you tell them the truth about things like that."

We had a couple beers and talked about aunts, uncles, and cousins. Then he gave me a ride back to my company area. As I got out of his jeep, we shook hands, he wished me luck with my tour, and thanked me for stopping by. He informed me that his time in the Army was almost at an end and that he was leaving in a couple of days for home.

After Michael drove away, I still felt overwhelmed. So, I tried talking with the chaplain. He advised me to pray but praying didn't make the horror go away. The gripping effect of my first few days in-country and the spell they cast over me blended into the shock of the new day's events. My sleep that night was interrupted by scenes of Billy and the grunts mixed with vignettes of me filling sandbags and swimming in breaking waves surrounded by dead bodies.

CHAPTER FIVE

By the end of my first week in-country, my luck took an unexpected turn breaking me away from the horror of the first few days. During roll call at company formation, the cherries received our permanent duty assignments.

My orders were to report to the 523rd Signal Battalion. As I left the mess hall after breakfast with the other cherries, I heard a familiar voice calling my name. I turned around and couldn't believe my eyes. A friendly face from back home caught me by surprise.

Danny Amato was sitting in a jeep, waving for me to come over and get in. I had grown up with him; he graduated from high school a year ahead of me and was drafted the year before me. I ran over, jumped into Danny's jeep, and grabbed his out-stretched hand.

He came from a large family. His younger brother, who had been in my high-school class was killed in a train wreck when we were seniors. I don't think Danny ever got over the loss. They were less than a year apart and looked like twins.

Every time I looked at Danny, I thought I was looking at Paul. They had both been great athletes during our years growing up. They were both the same height. If I stood next to them in line at school, I felt like a dwarf—me barely five-feet-eight inches and both of them a little over six feet. But sitting together in the jeep dressed in camouflaged fatigues and jungle boots, we were equals.

"I thought you joined the Navy. He said."

I gave him a short version of my Army/Navy story. When I was through talking, Danny took over the conversation.

"Well I'm a short timer. My tour in Vietnam is ending in a couple days. So, the captain gave me the duty of picking up new guys at the reception station, showing them around the base and dropping them at their duty stations."

"You mean this is just a coincidence. You didn't know I'd be here.?"

"Are you shitting me, or what? They just send new people to us at random to fill in jobs that have become vacant for all kinds of reasons: people killed in action, wounded, or rotated out for going home or being sent out to the bush."

"So, no one knows we're from the same hometown?"

"Not yet. But they will when I get you squared away with the first sergeant. But not only am I supposed to bring you to the 523rd Signal Battalion; I'm supposed to give you the grand tour of Chu Lai."

As we drove away from the reception station, we left a trail of dust behind us.

"Just another US military airbase," he said. "They're all over Southeast Asia fucking up the place."

I began to wonder what I was in for during his grand tour. But all of a sudden, he stopped the jeep: turned towards me and looked me directly in the eyes with such intensity it scared me.

"Don't let this place fuck you up."

Then he relaxed a bit.

"I'm sorry if I seem like I have a give-a-fuck attitude,

but most of us short-timers get that way. I hope to get rid of it before I get home."

He gave me a friendly punch to the shoulder.

"I just hope you make it home. This place is hell."

Danny took us on a utility road to the northern most point of the airbase. It was on a cliff jutting out over an inlet from the sea just barely inside a wire perimeter. When we got there, he stopped the jeep and pointed at the water below.

"You're looking at the brown-water Navy." He said. "It's where they dock Vietnam's version of PT Boats. We call them Swift Boats."

The area looked like the end of a man-made channel from the ocean dredged through a marshy tidal flat. I could see the swift boats, along with a variety of other US Navy vessels: Landing Ship Tanks, Armored Troop Carriers, and Cargo Vessels just to name a few.

Danny pointed to a string of coiled, razor-sharp barb-wire snaking its way along the marshy inland waterway that traveled in a southerly direction.

"You'll be pulling guard duty in the bunkers that make up that part of our defensive perimeter. It goes the whole length of the coastal plain, all the way to Highway One, and ends at the village of Anh Ton, which is right across the road from the main gate to Chu Lai."

He laughed a little and told me the village had all kinds of contraband for sale including marijuana and prostitutes He backed the jeep up and away from the edge of the cliff and continued with his grand tour.

"Our company area is about halfway to the village, but only the guard truck is allowed to drive on the perimeter road. Otherwise, I could drop you off at company headquarters, and give you a closer look at the bunker line on the way."

"What's guard duty like along our perimeter?" I asked.

"I've got to warn you: even though it looks like nobody can get through that wire, they do. Sapper squads have special training to penetrate the perimeter, and they get through in spite of the three layers of concertina-wire laced with tangle foot."

"What's tangle foot?" I asked.

"It's extra razor-sharp, zigzagging wire woven throughout the coils of concertina wire—the ugly coiled barbed wire. Sappers get through it anyway and plant satchel bombs."

"Satchel bombs?"

Danny laughed.

"Man, you really are a cherry. Satchel bombs are canvas bags full of explosives. They have straps attached to them, so the sappers can drag them through the wire as they go and use them to cause damage in all kinds of strategic locations inside this supposedly fortified area."

"Like what?"

"Those boats you saw at the brown-water Navy docks for one. The sappers blew a couple of them up not long ago. And over to our left, up on that ridgeline overhanging the beach, a helicopter pad was hit with rockets last week. No one was killed but a few guys were wounded. And those planes down in that crater to our right—that look like ghost ships—were blown up the night you flew in."

"I guess that's what we saw as we were landing."

"Probably was. And sappers go after communication bunkers, ammo bunkers, fuel dumps, and anything else they can crawl to at night. On their way in and out of the area, they try to silently sneak into our bunkers along the fence line you see in front of us, slit our throats, and escape without being seen. So, don't fall asleep in those bunkers."

We headed south on the main road of the airbase, stopping at an area along the shore.

"See those old wrecked buildings along this part of the beach? They were destroyed in a marine amphibious assault in 1965. It was kind of like the guys storming the beaches of Normandy in WWII."

A quick flash of my encounter there the day before ran through my mind. But I kept quiet.

We passed a sign identifying the Americal Division's Tactical Operations Center as DTOC. The Americal Division was officially the 23rd Infantry Division, otherwise known as the American, New Caledonian Division

Then he pulled the jeep up on to a knoll overlooking a mantle of pristine, soft, white sand bordered by the sea, waves breaking against the shore, with crisp sunshine, coconut palm trees, and a rocky coral reef. What a contrast with the sounds of war behind us.

"If you're lucky enough to find a board, you could go surfing out there," Danny said with a laugh. "Grunts use the beach when they come in from the bush for a stand down. But don't let them give you a hard time about having it easy because you're not out in the bush. They harass us and call us REMFs, and they have no idea what we do for our jobs."

I told Danny about me guarding Billy, and the situation he had with grunts.

"Doesn't that just burn your ass," he said. "The grunts think we have it easy in these communication bunkers. But they don't know anything about us. Let them operate our equipment through a shit storm some night and see how they like it."

We drove past some small airfields utilized for local-fire missions. Danny told me a little about the Navy Seabees constructing the runways for the landing of jet fighters by using a new development in combat airfield paving. He said they installed aluminum plank matting called AM-2. Since then, AM-2 has become the standard answer to the problems of airfield construction in combat zones. They claim it solves a lot of concerns about speed, placement, and versatility of use under the constant worry of wartime conditions.

When Danny finished telling me about the Seabees, he pulled the jeep up to a helicopter pad on a cliff next to a hospital—it was practically hanging over the ocean.

"Right down below, where you see all those antennas

sticking up in the air, is where your radio relay bunker is located. All the radio signals coming in from the bush go through that signal center."

"Really. Where do they go?"

"Some of them get converted to landlines—to let officers use telephones instead of radios in their air-conditioned vans."

"That sounds typical of the military."

"The rest of the signals are relayed from one field position to another and when the officers in the command bunkers make their decisions, their orders go back out to the bush. So, we are right in the middle of all the shit that is going on around the whole operational area."

"Are we safe in the signal bunker?"

"No. The gooks love hitting it with RPGs and 122-millimeter rockets, trying to knock out our communications to isolate everyone from each another. I'm sure you'll find out the hard way."

We moved on with our grand tour to the main gate along Highway One, the only paved road going north and south through the whole country. From there, he pointed out Landing Zone Hurricane, a fuel dump, and the main airfields of the Marine Aviation Groups, where planes take off carrying bombs to drop on Cambodia and North Vietnam.

Then, we passed by an ammo bunker, Landing Zone Bayonet, and a cave, which Danny said was used by the North Vietnamese Army at one time.

"So, there you have it," he said with another laugh. "Now you know your way around. Don't get lost."

We arrived at the 523rd Signal Battalion at about 1300 hours. Danny brought me to the headquarters building. It looked like most of the buildings around me, except it was twice the size of the rest. It had a door in the front with a small set of steps down to a gravel path and a door in the back with a gang plank for running out and into a bunker when under fire.

To the left of the headquarters building, the path continued running through the middle of a sprawling row of shacks laid out in a uniform pattern from east to west. All those structures were called hooches and appeared to be temporarily thrown together with 4x4 wood posts in the four corners of the flimsy shack. Plywood made up the lower sides of the walls and screens were used for the upper parts of the walls.

The roofs were made of corrugated tin with sandbags holding the roofs in place and adding protection to those inside. The hooches were where we slept. They had front doors opening to small porches and a back door with no porch and just a couple of steps down to another gravel wash that looked like the arroyos in a desert that drained the surrounding area during the rainy monsoon season.

When Danny introduced me to the First Sergeant, he was told he could catch a chopper at 1400 hours to Cam Rahn Bay and fly home the next day. We gave each other bear hugs and wished each other well.

That was the last I saw of Danny Amato. By the time I got home from Vietnam, Danny was dead. He had slit his own throat.

A Long Triage

CHAPTER SIX

After I presented my identification papers and orders to the First Sergeant, he issued me an assortment of personal supplies including an M16 assault rifle and several clips of ammunition. Then he told me to report to Specialist Fourth Class Jared Pasquale at A Company in hooch number five.

"He's a little red-headed guy, and he is the senior man in the hooch. He'll assign you to a bunk. you're dismissed."

I saluted and said, "Yes Sergeant." And stepped out of the headquarters' building.

As I walked around the company area on my own, like a lost puppy, looking for hooch number five, I could see some of the places Danny had shown me from his jeep on our grand tour of the base. I walked across the small airfields he said were used for local fire missions. Heavy aluminum matting had been laid on the ground and the different sections were joined together by metal connectors with special mats, forming a centerline that had catapults and guide rails for the planes when they were taking off and landing. For a moment, I felt like I was standing on the deck of an aircraft carrier, except concertina wire and sandbagged bunkers along the perimeter surrounded me instead of the ocean.

When I Finally found hooch number five, I could see Jared sitting out front on the porch waiting for me to arrive. He looked as though he was a couple years older than me. He was short and thin with flaming-red hair and appeared to have a wiry strength about him. A sharp wit and certain intelligence were evident when he spoke.

"So, you're our new cherry," he said as we shook hands. "Private Sullivan from Massachusetts, I've been told. Welcome to the war. I'm Jared from Milwaukee, Wisconsin."

"Nice to meet you Jared from Milwaukee. I'm Kerry from Sandy Cove."

"Just so you know right from the start, I didn't want to be in this fucking war. I enlisted in the Army to escape a bum rap with the law back home.

"What happened?"

"I was the designated driver one night when my friends trashed the town with graffiti and knocked over mailboxes for the fun of it. I didn't even help them do it. But they were all juveniles. So, they got off easy. Because I was over eighteen, I was legally the only adult and the judge held me responsible for the whole mess."

"That sucks," I said.

"Yeah it does. And to make matters worse, the DA told the judge that I was trying to dodge the draft. So, he gave me a choice between being charged with a crime or joining the Army. And if I made it home from Vietnam, he said he would dismiss the case. So, here I am. What's your story?"

"I was in the process of joining the Navy, but one of my friends dodged the draft and I was next on the list to fill our town's quota for the month of March. So, when I reported to the Boston Army base for my pre-induction physical, they scooped me up, put me on a bus, and sent me to Fort Dix in New Jersey for basic training, and then to Fort Gordon, Georgia, for signal school. When my training was completed, they gave me a thirty-day leave and then shipped me over here."

****

As we entered the hooch, Jared said, "This is a bummer Sully, but you might as well know why a bunk is available in our hooch. A few days before you got here, me and Zebra Man were sent out to LZ Green Haven to operate the mobile radio van while the regular crew went on R&R. But he didn't make it back with me."

I felt horrible hearing this. I said nothing as I walked in and saw a group of guys sitting around passing a pipe to one another.

His friends, who had all been in-country for about six months, were in the middle of an improvised requiem ceremony in his honor. Apparently, Zebra Man had been a pot smoker. As they passed around the pot pipe, each person took a hit and said a few words of respect and remembrance. When Jared got the pipe, he held it for a long time and gave the eulogy.

He began by saying, "Carlos Encinias was his name, but he was Zebra Man to us."

He took a drag from the pipe before continuing. "He lived in New Mexico before joining the Army right out of high school. He served in the Korean War and was older than the rest of us enlisted men here in Vietnam, but he was our soul mate. We called him Zebra Man because he earned and lost his sergeant stripes many times—protecting us from poor decisions made by the officers who live and work in those air-conditioned vans, surrounding their big important command-control bunker. All while we sweat like pigs sleeping under nets hiding from mosquitoes." He paused for a moment of silence.

I looked around the room, taking note of where everything was. On both sides of the center aisle, there were four sections clearly separated by their contents. From front to back, each area had a bunk beneath a metal frame holding up a mosquito net. A standard olive-green metal footlocker sat on the floor next to the bunk. There was a passageway in the middle of the area separating the locker and the bunk from a tall standing locker at the end. Pictures of family and friends were taped to the lockers along with a few Playboy pinup posters and sports paraphernalia. I was impressed with how clean the place looked considering it was occupied by eight young men.

When the moment of silence ended, Jared continued with the eulogy. "Zebra Man's last and final effort to protect his men should earn him the medal of honor. We were sent out to the bush to help a group of South Vietnamese soldiers strengthen their defenses on a hill, a hill we all knew was a lost cause. It had been taken and abandoned many times by both sides of this useless war. The firebase was on high alert and scouts were out observing enemy-troop movements in the valley below."

Jared paused again; he appeared to be shaking a little as he wiped away tears running over his cheeks. His voice crackled as he went on to say, "Before dawn on the day Zebra Man was killed, three infantry soldiers were outside the perimeter on a helicopter pad below us. We began taking small-arms fire. Zebra Man sent me to pack the radios and prepare the van to be airlifted off the hill, so the gooks wouldn't get the equipment."

Jared wiped another tear and continued. "The gooks appeared on the hill above us and began a downward assault with automatic weapons, rockets, and mortars. Shrapnel was showering down on all of us. I finished packing the van, jumped in and was ready for the airlift. Zebra Man screamed to the three grunts, 'Run for the van and jump in, I'll set the hook for the airlift.' The grunts ran like hell, jumped into the van with me, the helicopter swooped in, and Zebra Man leapt through the air. As he set the hook, he was shot in the back by a sniper. His body fell to the ground as the chopper flew away with me and the grunts safely inside."

After hearing such a story, I didn't dare refuse the invitation to join the ceremony. As Jared finished, he passed the pipe to me and said, "Welcome to Vietnam, Sully. You never met Zebra Man, but I'm sure he would appreciate a few words of respect from the cherry taking over his bunk."

"God rest your soul, Zebra Man," then I took my very first hit of marijuana. I passed the pipe to the guy next to me. A daze covered me like a blanket of fog: I started coughing and tried to sit down slowly. I somehow stumbled to my new bunk and passed out.

****

In the morning, Jared had to shake me awake. "Sully, you missed company formation. But don't worry; I covered for you with the captain. He told me to show you around the battalion area and give you an orientation." We made some small talk about back home and our families.

Then he got serious and said, "When your paperwork is cleared, you'll start regular shifts at A Company's signal center. Your primary job will be to operate and maintain radio terminals from 1800 to 0600. The main channels connect the landing zones, firebases, and infantry companies out in the bush with each other and to DTOC. The order wire is reserved for communication between the operators for maintenance purposes and emergency situations."

He paused for a moment and then said, "You got that?"

I gave a nod, and Jared went on. "The captain said you were trained to operate the circuit control boards. Here in the Nam we call them patch panels. The system allows the officers in their air-conditioned vans to have the convenience of using telephones instead of radios. Only a few guys have that training. So, even when it's not your shift, unless you're out on the bunker line, you'll need to get to the signal center during shit storms."

I asked, "Are we going in there today?"

He said, "Only to show you around and meet some of the other guys. Don't worry. You'll be working in there soon enough. And eventually when the rockets and mortars start coming in, you'll wish you could get out of there because you'll feel like a sitting duck. But before you start pulling shifts in there, you'll probably spend some time on details: burning shit, pulling KP, guard duty, and maybe even a turn with C Company to see what goes on out in the field."

All the equipment was housed in green metal cargo vans which could be mounted on trucks or trailers, and, if necessary, airlifted by helicopter. However, in this case the vans were mostly buried underground along with a variety of other equipment with antennas protruding through the roofline.

Jared said, "We call this place our underground radio station."

It looked more like a mausoleum buried in the ground, completely covered over with sandbags arranged in an overlapping brick like pattern with a rabbit burrow for an entryway.

Jared said, "Once you start working a regular shift with us, in addition to your duties at the signal center, every fourth night you'll rotate out of the signal center and into one of the bunkers along the perimeter for guard duty. The rotating schedule allows someone else to rotate into the signal center to replace you on those nights." He paused and said, "You know, man, share and share alike."

Like all signalmen, I had been trained to perform my duties during nuclear, chemical, biological, radiological, and conventional warfare, as well as counterinsurgency. My work included, but was not limited to, installation, operation, and maintenance of the radio and circuit-control equipment assigned to me. In order to accomplish our missions, the commanders established Standing Operational Procedures, or SOPs, as routine combat orders to avoid the necessity of repeating instructions to everyone, especially when engaged with the enemy. These procedures were unique to each unit, and not to be confused with Standard Army Protocols, or SAPs, which are primarily generic and geared toward peacetime operations.

Unfortunately, when under direct- or indirect-enemy fire, or even friendly fire, sometimes this dichotomy brought individual soldiers reacting to horrific unexpected emergency circumstances into direct conflict with the chain of command, resulting in unnecessary tragedy, and, in some cases, unfair disciplinary actions similar to the case of Billy and the grunts.

At lunchtime, Jared said, "Go back to our hooch, square away your area, and meet me at the mess hall at 1300 hours. I've got to report to the captain."

Again, I felt like that lost puppy. My living space was

in the company area on the opposite side of the airstrips and helicopter pads from the signal center. My hooch was a shack mounted on a wooden platform, 20 feet by 32 feet, with a corrugated tin roof held in place by sandbags. The sides were screened in with roll down canvas flaps for use during windy and rainy times, mostly monsoon season. Screen doors were in the center at both ends of the rectangular hut.

The areas running parallel between the hooches were partially dugout with metal drainage culverts, half buried and covered over with sandbags perched strategically for protection during the rocket and mortar attacks that everyone was calling shit storms.

During lunch, Jared had to reintroduce me to my hooch mates because I couldn't remember their names from the night before. My failing memory provided them with some fun, joking about my being a cherry and a newly inducted member of the pot smokers of Chu Lai.

After lunch Jared showed me more of the company area and introduced me to more of the guys I would be working with at the signal center and sharing guard duty with out on the bunker line.

He said, "Every day, unless I CORP is hot with enemy activity, the captain insists that people who are not on duty during the daylight hours participate in PT—you know, physical training. If the area is hot with enemy action, then he insists that the troops not bunch up in groups, in order to avoid giving the gooks tempting targets. So, when it's hot, there's no PT or hanging around bunched up in groups for playing ball or anything else."

On this particular day, the area was not hot with enemy action, but the temperature was around 100° Fahrenheit. Those of us not on duty were ordered to report to the basketball court.

Jared said the court was the remains of a cement slab that had been the floor of a command bunker. The bunker was blown to bits by 122-mm rockets during the Tet Offensive that year, but the slab remained intact. When we got to the court, he pointed to a screen door sitting up in a tree and said, "That's all that's left of that poor old command bunker after all the explosions. We leave the door up there to remind us not to take quiet times for granted and to always be alert."

When we formed up on the basketball court, our captain was there to greet us. He said, "We are privileged to have Marines from the Republic of Korea with us today. They have agreed to give you people a refresher course in self-defense. Give them your undivided attention and cooperation." Then he left the area.

The three Koreans looked battle worn and fierce with bands of human ears hanging from their belts. Their ghastly image freaked me out. I felt like I was one of the naïve wimpy characters stuck in some old black-and-white Vincent Price horror movie, ready to run and hide someplace safe.

When they spoke in broken English, it sounded like gibberish to me. But they also gestured with hand signals and grabbed me and two other cherries with painful wrist locks and moved us into a position with our backs tightly circling the pole holding up the basketball net, and then tied sandbags around the pole directly over our heads.

They made it clear by use of threatening motions and screaming in our faces that they were going to attack us with full contact karate blows to our bodies, and that we needed to defend ourselves or we would be injured. The three of them paused for a moment, bowed respectfully with their hands held in prayer position, stood directly face to face with us and shouted, "he-a-a-ah-now!"

Before I could do anything at all, or even had a chance to defend myself, the man in front of me jumped up in the air, kicked the sandbag with his bare foot, and landed safely back in the position he started from. Sand began to trickle down the back of my neck. "Unbelievable," I whispered quietly to myself. "You've got to be kidding me." A lot of drama without much action. The refresher course continued. Despite the language and cultural barrier and some odd techniques, we did learn valuable self-defense techniques that afternoon.

After the course was dismissed, Jared and the rest of

my hooch mates met at the mess hall for supper. They grilled me with questions about myself, and when I ran out of things to say they told their own stories.

Jake, the tallest of the crew, was from Detroit Michigan. He said, "I was drafted after graduating from college. I'm almost glad it happened. I'd been dating the same girl all through those four years. I liked her a lot, but she was ready to get married and I wasn't. But maybe if I had gotten married and had kids like she wanted, I could have avoided Vietnam."

He had come over to Vietnam on the same plane as Jared. They were both telephone switchboard operators and worked at the signal center. When they stood side by side, they looked like the cartoon characters Mutt and Jeff.

Cheeseman went next. "I'm from California and I enlisted to get out of South-Central LA. If I hadn't, I would have been killed or killed someone else. The gangs run the streets and I wanted nothing to do with them. At least if I get killed in the Nam, my family will think I'm a hero."

He also told me he was one of the guys who ran the diesel generators that provided electricity for the signal center. He had the barrel chest and thick muscular build of a weightlifter.

When Cheeseman finished talking, Levi took over the

conversation. He was from Tennessee and the most serious looking one of the group. Short like me but thick and solid all around, he worked as one of the pole jockeys maintaining the landlines running around the base along with a crew of other guys. He was an Army brat, raised with his brother and sister all over the world on the military bases where his father was stationed.

Larry, a tall skinny character, was a draftee and drove the potable water truck around the Americal Division, making sure we always had enough drinking water. Before being drafted, he lived in Connecticut in the summers and Florida in the winter with his parents, who were retired teachers.

Andy, about the same shape and size as me, was from Texas. He had been drafted right out of high school and worked in the motor pool. He was a gifted mechanic. His family owned a large trucking company, and he started learning the trade from an early age.

After supper, those of us who were not on duty were allowed the freedom to roam around the base without supervision to visit friends, play cards, read, go to the enlisted men's club . . . whatever our choice. But Jared said to me, "You need to report to the captain after breakfast in the morning. So, get a good night's sleep. You never know what to expect from him."

CHAPTER SEVEN

I had been in Vietnam for barely a week, and I already had orders to report to the company commander. I was a nervous wreck. I had no idea why he would want to see me. I hadn't done anything that could possibly have gotten me into trouble. So, I was determined to hold my ground and handle whatever was coming my way.

Without hesitation, I walked up the two steps of the porch in the front of the little plywood building and knocked firmly on the screen door to his office.

"Good morning Captain. Private Sullivan reporting as ordered, Sir,"

"Enter, and stand at ease," was his reply.

As I entered and took the proper military position, I was surprised at how young he appeared to be, baby faced with blonde hair—longer than I expected for an officer. His office was picture perfect, a place for everything and everything in its place: military manuals in alphabetical order, weapons neatly organized, rifles on his left, and pistols on his right.

"Just call me Captain. You've been here, what . . . about a week?"

"Today's my seventh day, if you count the night I landed, Captain."

"According to your papers, you went to jump school and were supposed to become an airborne ranger."

"No, Captain, that's not accurate."

"Then why have I got orders here telling me to send you over to the Recondo School instead of assigning you to the signal bunker."

I had no idea why he would be asking me a question like that. And I figured my luck was about to go downhill.

"What's Recondo School, Captain?"

"It's a three week in-country training program to prepare you for LLRPs, you know Long Range Reconnaissance Patrol. But you're supposed to have already been trained as a paratrooper before you go there."

"I thought you had to volunteer to go to jump school."

"You must have signed yourself up for something during basic training or signal school, because here are the orders."

"But Captain, I didn't."

With pursed lips and a confused and frustrated look on his baby face, he began shuffling papers around on his shiny, new olive-green metal desk. After a few minutes, he seemed to give up trying to understand what he was reading and turned to me.

"Well, the way I see it, you've got three options."

"What would they be?"

"You can report to the Recondo School as ordered and just follow more orders. They have an in-country jump school there for new guys."

"Sorry captain, but I'm not interested."

"Or, you could accept a non-judicial disciplinary action, called an article fifteen, for not following orders."

"With all due respect, Captain, I'm not taking an article fifteen. I haven't done anything wrong."

"Then we're stuck with option number three. You'll stay here in the company area, burning shit, pulling KP, and having guard duty until we straighten things out."

He squinted his eyes and gave me another perplexed look of indignation.

So, there I was, just a week into my yearlong tour of duty in America's unjust and unpopular war. I'm a scared shitless cherry, I already have a serious resentment toward this REMF and grunt bullshit, and now my orders are screwed up.

My inner voice started tormenting me, "Typical institutional hypocrisy that happens all the time, screwing things up, bullies pushing you around and messing with your head. You don't even believe in this stupid war."

It wasn't right and I wanted to do something about it. But I had to remain calm. I was afraid the Captain would think I was a wimp or, worse, crazy—talking to myself, and have me sent home on a section eight psychiatric discharge. I knew I needed to get hold of myself and come to terms with the events of my first week in-country.

After a long pause, I asked the captain if I could have some time to think about what I wanted to do before I made a decision.

He said, "I'll put you on hold-over status until we get your orders straightened out. Go ahead and take a few hours off, but report for guard duty at 1600. I'll place you on company details for now; you might as well be of some use while we wait."

"Yes, Captain. Where do I report for guard duty?"

"Right next to the water tank. You can't miss it. I'll let First Sergeant know you start perimeter guard tonight. You're dismissed."

****

After I left the captains office, I roamed around the company area for the rest of the morning and part of the afternoon. For future reference, I located the Vietnamese laundry out behind the Captain's office. Then I walked over to the motor pool and looked around just to kill some time. I was fascinated by what I saw out behind the buildings: trucks, armored personnel carriers, communication vans—and they all looked like they had been hit by explosive devices and were burned beyond recognition.

After I left the junkyard, I went over to the mess hall for lunch. I sat down with some of the guys in the company that I didn't know yet and asked a lot of questions about my situation. Their answers varied from "Tough shit" to "Fuck'em all—lifers don't know what they're doing anyway. So, suck it up, be a man, and just do what you're told."

"Thanks a lot guys."

****

After I left the mess hall and went back to my hooch, I laid down on my bunk, and fell asleep. About an hour later someone came through the hooch calling out for those of us who had guard duty to get our asses in gear and make it to guard formation over by the water tank immediately.

I grabbed my gear, ran over to the water tank, and just made it to the formation in time for my name to be called by the sergeant in charge of the bunkers out on the perimeter surrounding the base. I fell in line.

"Right here, Sergeant."

He checked my weapon, ammunition pouches, eyeballed my uniform, and said, "Not bad for a cherry."

We were ordered to load the guard truck with a variety of ammo boxes. Some contained extra rounds for our M16s, some contained flares, and some contained grenades.

Before we climbed aboard, the sergeant said, "Seeing that we have a few cherries here today, I'll give a short review."

He paused for a moment and looked around to make sure we were all paying attention to him. When he was satisfied, he went on with his review.

"For obvious reasons, bullets, flares, and grenades are stored in separate ammo boxes. Any questions?"

No response from anybody.

"Only use flares to light up the area if you suspect the enemy is attempting to penetrate the perimeter. If he is, it's probably sappers trying to crawl through the wire. It takes them so long to get through, you'll have time to call DTOC on your field phone."

He paused again and looked around eyeballing the cherries, like we were idiots.

"Only throw grenades if you receive confirmation from an officer that we are in fact having an attempted penetration of the perimeter."

Several short timers complained.

"That's bullshit Sarge. We need to defend ourselves anyway we can."

"You guys know you don't need to call in for permission to shoot the enemy with your rifles if you actually see the fuckers. . . at all times defend yourselves with your M16s."

****

As the sergeant's review was coming to an end, out of the corner of my eye, I could see one of the guys climbing into the truck. He must have been a cherry like me because his hair was still in a military crew cut and his uniform was pressed and spotless. I figured like me, it must be his first time going out to the bunker line. I never did get his name. But he made a lasting impression on me that continues to haunt me.

I could sense something wasn't quite right; he was fidgeting with the ammo boxes and squinting his eyes in the sun while staring at something he had in his hands—like he had never seen the stuff before. As it turned out, he had a couple ammo cans open and was looking through them.

I heard the sergeant of the guard scream at him, "You idiot! Put those things down." The guy stopped immediately, and the sergeant made him do some push-ups and finish loading the truck with supplies by himself.

The rest of us started loading our personal gear and began climbing into the truck. But I heard a sizzling sound as I was about to sit down and give a helping hand to one of the other guys. He must have heard the same noise. He had a frightful look on his face as he pulled me backwards with a tight grip on my wrist and yelled, "Jump!"

As most of us jumped out of the truck and landed flat ass in the dirt, an extremely loud explosion went off like a bomb. Shattered truck parts flew through the smoke-filled air, landing all around us, and an unmerciful screaming vibrated through the atmosphere.

I turned and looked. I couldn't believe what I saw. I was grossed out and felt like throwing up. The cherry that had loaded the truck was now missing the lower parts of both legs.

A couple of short-timers, both experienced infantry soldiers, had the wherewithal to grab their web belts and apply tourniquets to both legs on the wounded soldier. The rest of the cherries stood around dumbstruck, waiting for the sergeant to tell us what to do.

We were in a state of shock with squeamish, puke-ready looks on our faces but afraid to say anything in front of the experienced short-timers. We were fearful of the dreaded question, "What are you, a REMF?"

The sergeant got on his radio and called for the medics. When he was through, he lectured us about the consequences of making stupid mistakes.

He said, "That dummy must have mixed flares and grenades in the same ammo box. One of the caps on the flares probably loosened and ignited—setting off the grenades."

As shocking and unsettling as the experience was, we had a job to do. We hiked over to the motor pool, requisitioned another truck, and got it loaded with troops, equipment, and ammunition.

The sergeant of the guard drove us along the utility road Danny had shown me during our grand tour of Chu Lai. We arrived at the bunker line before dark to relieve the guys who had been on daytime guard duty. Only two guys per bunker were on duty for day guard. As we picked them up, we were dropped off in groups of three for night guard.

Welcome to My War

****

Ground-level bunkers were soggy, foul, and rat-infested. Some were partially dug into the surrounding landscape. 4x4 wood posts held up tin roofs covered by sandbags forming a square big enough for two Army cots on opposite sides of the back wall, with an opening between them for a person to enter or exit. A rick-rack pattern of sandbags made up the remainder of the walls but left space for observation and room to fire your weapon when you needed to.

At strategic intervals along the perimeter—about every fourth or fifth defensive position—a sandbagged platform was perched upon a tower like the crow's nest on large sailing vessels. Field phones connected each bunker to the immediate left and right and were daisy chained by telephone wire around the base, connecting all the bunkers to a command center.

Every night a non-commissioned officer was required to stay awake at company headquarters. He was the acting commander while the captain got his sleep. We referred to him as the CQ—charge of quarters.

An enlisted man was always assigned to do the legwork. We called him the CQ runner. Only the enlisted men were assigned to man the ground level bunkers along the perimeter. And an NCO was stationed in every tower. In this way, the area was considered secure for the night.

****

Geographically, the war in Vietnam was not like other wars. It was not concentrated along an identifiable frontline that moved as one side lost and the winning side gained territory. Instead, it was fought in patches and strips of North Vietnamese communist-held positions that were spread all around South Vietnam amongst the villages and rice paddies of the civilian population and deep in the jungle.

On a map, the American and South Vietnamese installations looked like squares on a quilt, spread throughout the countryside, and along the coastline. Defensive bunkers and concertina-wire perimeters surrounded each enclave. Terrorist attacks on our positions, mostly at night, were frequent and intended to encourage us to pack up and leave.

It seemed like something spooky happened every time I was out on the bunker line. There were mountains surrounding us on three sides, with marshland and rice paddies scattered around the coastal plains between the foothills and the perimeter wire. Little rivers flowed out of the marshland and into the South China Sea on the fourth side.

Quite frequently, the tops of the mountains appeared

to lift up into the sky during thunderous strikes when B-52s dropped bombs throughout the night. Those images still haunt me, especially on the Fourth of July. But I have to admit it was quite a show.

The United States had great names for these air campaigns: Rolling Thunder, Barrel Roll, and Arc Light Strikes. But a serious loss of aircraft caused Secretary of Defense Robert McNamara to reactivate the USS New Jersey, a decommissioned battleship from the days of World War II.

The giant ship was stationed along our coastline for several months delivering payloads of explosives upon enemy positions throughout the country. Her massive guns were sixteen inches in diameter and fired 2,700-pound shells up to twenty-three miles away. This may have sounded great to the commanders, but to us poor bastards sitting in the bunkers below, it was a living nightmare. While we heard what sounded like explosive freight trains whistling over our heads as the shells flew through the air, we prayed the damn things didn't fall short of their targets and land on top of us.

The New Jersey was the only active battleship in the world at the time. Her crew was extremely effective during her redeployment. They fired close to twenty-thousand rounds during her time off the coast of Vietnam. Her firepower sank enemy logistical vessels before they could reach the beaches. Nothing within her range was safe from destruction. She inflicted heavy damage to motor vehicles carrying enemy troops and supplies, and she eliminated concrete observation towers, enemy caves, and many other strategic targets.

But what amazed me the most, aside from the Arc Light Strikes or the New Jersey firing from the off-shore coastal gun-line, was the resilience of the Viet Cong and the North Vietnamese Regular Army. The morning after a brutal shelling, surviving enemy soldiers would crawl out from all the devastation, clean up the area as best they could, and be ready to fight another day."

CHAPTER EIGHT

It took the captain a few weeks to straighten out my paperwork. During that time, I remained on holdover status and continued to be assigned a variety of company details: shit-burning detail, KP, or guard duty. There was a series of explosions inside our perimeter behind our bunker on one of the nights that I was on guard duty.

When the explosions stopped, we could hear alarms screeching and men shouting. Some were shouting orders; some were shouting in pain. Then I heard somebody shout, "Charlie, we're going to kill you and your whole fucking family." And then secondary explosions blew off several moments later—probably fuel and ammunition at the storage depots.

All three of us in my bunker knew it could only mean one thing. Someone had fallen asleep and sappers had gotten through the wire.

I can't speak for anybody else, but I felt like I was going to have a heart attack. My breathing became labored, my heart was pounding rapidly, and I began to sweat profusely. I was in a state of panic. We didn't dare take turns sleeping. So, we chattered nervously for the rest of the night to keep each other awake.

The next morning, the guard truck was running late. We got a little edgy while waiting for it to arrive. We knew something wasn't quite right. When the guard truck finally arrived with the day guards, the shock of seeing three bodies laid out in the bed of the truck made me puke. Their throats were slit wide open, and their bodies were stripped bare. Even their dog tags were missing. The truck was late because it took quite a bit of time to clean up the mess.

The dead guys had been on guard duty in the bunker, just down the line to the left of ours. Performing the same job as us. The sergeant, a gung-ho infantryman himself, said, "See what happens when you fall asleep on guard duty? Let this be a lesson to all you REMFs—don't let your buddies fall asleep in these bunkers when the alert status is red." I never forgot.

On my last day of holdover status, I was on guard duty during daylight hours with Ronnie, a guy I had just met but heard of. The alert status was white, the lowest level of possible threat. So, I wasn't too concerned. Only one of the two guys in the bunker was required to maintain the watch. The other guy was allowed to write letters or read a book.

When my turn at the watch was over, I told Ronnie I was going to read for a while. He said, "Sure, man, I got it covered." But he didn't have it covered.

I was leaning against the post in the front corner of the bunker reading. Suddenly, I felt a sting on the tip of my earlobe. I thought it was a bee. I tried to slap it away but as I looked up, I heard the crack of gunfire. I saw a Viet Cong soldier in the marshy grass, taking aim at me, and getting ready to fire a second shot. Ronnie returned fire and the guy disappeared into the swampy waters of the marsh.

When the field-phone rang, Ronnie answered. He reported that he accidentally fired his weapon. Then he turned to me and said, "Sorry, man, I dozed off a little. But the bastard's gone now and won't be back for the rest of the day. If I told Sarge what really happened, one of us would get in a lot of trouble for falling asleep. Do me a favor and let's keep it to ourselves. I'm leaving in a week."

Not only did I have goose bumps for the rest of the day from the fear I felt, I was angry with him. But Ronnie was one of the popular guys in the company. I did the only thing I thought I could do. I kept my mouth shut and let the guy finish out his time in-country and go home. If I hadn't, I would have been black balled even by the guys I thought were my friends. As he finished up his last week, he told the other guys that I could be counted on and to back me up if the lifers gave me a hard time.

****

After several weeks of burning shit with gasoline, peeling potatoes, scrubbing pots and pans while on KP at the mess hall, and having guard duty out on the bunker line, the captain finally called me back into his office to deal with the problems related to my orders. When I entered, he said, "Private Sullivan, there doesn't have to be a court-martial or an article fifteen or any other kind of disciplinary action, if you and I can come to an agreement."

Although I was nervous and angry about my predicament, I responded calmly, "Yes, sir, I'll do my best to cooperate."

Then he said, "First, we need to get a few things straight between us. And if we do, you can start your regular shifts at the signal center tonight. It turns out you were right about the papers you signed back in the states."

He handed me copies of them and some personnel reports and said, "You can read these on your own time. I'll just summarize them for now. If it's all true, you could sign this form I have right here, and we can both move on without further delay."

"It sounds good to me so far, Captain."

He proceeded, "The reports say that during your basic training at Fort Dix New Jersey, you volunteered to attend a recruitment assembly held by the US Army Airborne School out of Fort Benning Georgia. When the assembly was over, you signed a form stating that you were interested in attending phase two of airborne orientation. The paper you signed specifically said it was not a final commitment to volunteer for airborne training. It was only a commitment to attend phase two of the recruitment orientation."

"Yes, Captain, that's the way I remember it."

"After you graduated from signal school at Fort Gordon Georgia, a personnel clerk messed up your orders and instead of sending you to Fort Benning for phase two, he sent you home on the automatic thirty-day leave everybody was getting before being shipped to Vietnam. When you got back from leave, they put you on holdover status pending your attendance at phase two."

"I tried to straighten it all out. But they wouldn't listen to me."

"Problem was, Private Sullivan, you told the airborne recruiter that you changed your mind because, while you were on leave, you learned that airborne radiomen are prime targets for enemy snipers when they jump out of planes and helicopters with the radio on their backs and that out in the bush a big whip antenna sticks up in the air making them an easy target.

The recruiter basically says that when you heard that, you chickened out. Then they sent you over here. So, you're off the hook. You never did officially volunteer for jump school."

The captain laughed a little and went on to say, "That explains why you landed here out of rotation with your classmates from signal school. Meanwhile, I've taken the liberty to have a new set of orders drawn up for you. The only problem is that I need you at the signal center for a complete yearlong tour of duty. That would extend your time in Vietnam beyond the mandatory twelve months. So, you would have to waive your current DEROS."

"What's DEROS, Captain?"

"It's the Army's acronym for Date Estimated for Return from Overseas. In other words, I can't make you stay here longer than twelve months unless you volunteer to do it."

"So, what do you want me to do?"

"I need your cooperation so the rotations of personnel will fall back into the SOPs I have to operate by. I just lost Encinias and Amato rotated out. I'm looking ahead for the needs of the company. If you'll sign the papers to volunteer to do the extra time in Vietnam, I'll make sure battalion approves your new orders. And the problem will be solved for both of us. As an added incentive, you'll be qualified for the early-out program and be discharged when you get stateside."

"What's the early-out program, Captain?"

"When soldiers return home from Vietnam with less than one hundred and fifty days left in the service before their ETS, they are discharged. ETS stands for expiration of term of service. In other words, it's your date of discharge."

"Why do they do that?"

"The powers that be, back home, have decided that draftees aren't worth keeping in the Army once you get home from Vietnam unless you have more than that amount of time left in the service. They figure you're too messed up in the head to bother with."

I had already heard about the early-out program, but I wanted to hear it from my captain for verification. A few days before the captain offered me this opportunity, I had received a letter from Billy who told me that he received an early out because he had less than one hundred and fifty days until his date of discharge when he got stateside. Other than the early out, I found the remainder of Billy's letter depressing.

In his letter he said, "Sully, the company officers transferred my witnesses to different units, and they were not available to testify about what really happened. My appointed attorney arranged a plea bargain and I accepted it. I plead to negligent homicide: no jail time and a general discharge with full veteran's benefits. And because I had less than one hundred and fifty days left before my discharge date, they wanted to get rid of me anyway. I was just glad to be out of the Army and done with all the bullshit."

With that in mind, I said, "With all due respect, Captain, I resent the characterization of me being chicken. The truth is I feel cheated. I was supposed to be in the Navy to begin with, but the draft board put me in the Army instead."

I actually wanted to be a paratrooper. I've always wanted to give jump school a try. But when I realized this war was not justified, I couldn't see taking extra chances with my life if I'm not fighting for a cause I believe in—just to prove myself in some macho way to people like that captain, the recruiters, or anybody else that thinks like that.

I took the forms and signed, but said, "Captain, I'm signing because you said when I'm done here, not only can I go home, I'll be able to get out of the Army early. I've about had it with the Army anyway."

He said, "I don't care about your reasons for signing, so long as you sign."

After I signed the forms, the captain said, "Private Sullivan, you've made a smart decision. An extra month in Vietnam will look good on your record. And getting out of the Army early is the best thing for you draftees, unless you change your mind and decide to stay in the service for a career. And if you do, you can always re-enlist when the time comes."

"Anything else, captain?"

"No, you're all set for now. Report to Sergeant DeCoste at the signal center at 1800 hours. You're dismissed until then."

I saluted and said, "Yes, Captain."

****

Inside I was pissed off. I had been in Vietnam for several weeks and had to start my twelve months in-country all over again or be tied up in some sort of disciplinary action. At least I finally had a permanent assignment. And I was happy to know I'd be getting out of the Army when I got home from Vietnam.

A Long Triage

CHAPTER NINE

I left the captain's office around lunchtime. But our conversation had ruined my appetite. I made my way back to the beach. I was pleasantly surprised to find the Chu Lai USO located there. Of course, I had to share the beach with a group of grunts in from the bush for stand down. I was a little paranoid about interacting with them because of my experience guarding Billy, as well as overhearing a lot of talk about grunts being better than REMFs. But I hung around and went swimming and surfing with some of them.

They had a serious amount of pot and wanted to share generously. I didn't dare flat out refuse, knowing it would have been taken as an insult and started a confrontation about REMFs and grunts. So, I politely thanked them for the offer and explained that I would be manning the communications for the night. I told them that I wouldn't want to fuck-up any relays and get anybody out in the bush killed. They seemed to like that reason and said they appreciated my attitude.

We had a great time for a couple of hours, and I left on good terms with them. I arrived at the signal center at 1750, crawled through the sandbagged rabbit hole of an entrance, stood up in the well-lit underground grotto, and met head on with a typical staff sergeant: big, thickly built, scowl-faced, cigar-smoking, and angry. He introduced himself as Sergeant DeCoste. Then he introduced me to an enlisted man he called Monty.

Sergeant DeCoste said, "Private Sullivan, I don't know what the captain told you, but I don't stick around here after 1800 unless there's an emergency. Monty will fill you in on what you need to know. For tonight, just shadow him while he does his work. You'll catch on soon enough."

Monty was another 19-year-old draftee. His real name was Randy Olson. He was born and raised in New York, but his family moved to Montpelier, Vermont, just before he was drafted. He was a little taller than me, about five feet ten inches in height, and a little overweight with blonde hair unexpectedly long for the Army.

He said, "I complained so much during basic training about hating my family's move that when the guys saw me, they would automatically say, 'We know, man,

Montpelier sucks and you wish you were in New York.' So, they started calling me Monty, just to bust my balls. The name stuck and followed me over here. And I hate this place, too."

The underground communication vans were arranged around a cement slab, laid out in a rectangle, with their doors missing and all facing into the center. In this way, soldiers could move in and out of each other's workspaces freely, and cover for each other when the occasion arose—which was mostly when under attack by enemy fire.

At the end of the rectangle opposite the main entryway, there was an empty van with no door and the back panel removed. It functioned as a tunnel separating the radio relays and patch panel from an area with switchboards and teletype equipment, which, according to rumor, reached all the way to Washington DC. You needed a security clearance to enter that back room. Evidently secret stuff went on in there.

Monty said, "Don't bother talking to the closed-lipped, tight-ass bastards who come and go through that tunnel. If you just say *hello*, they'll report you for breaching security so fast you won't know what happened and you'll wake up in the stockade."

For the next year, I worked the night shift at the signal center and didn't hear any secrets or have any problems with the guys in the back room. I spent most of my time at the signal center performing routine relays, connecting the infantry guys in the bush, landing zones, and firebases, with each other and to DTOC when they called for support from their commanders.

Eventually I got used to the nightly rockets and mortars dropping out of the sky and exploding on top of us while we worked the equipment and communicated with the other radio operators. We worked underground while the earth above us was rumbling and splitting apart from an earthquake.

During the shit storms, the first sound I could hear was a faint reverberating noise in the distance, like a subway train headed our way. Then a sound, almost like the explosion of crashing motor vehicles would sound closer, pounding and shaking the earth more violently than the first but from half the distance away, and a third explosion like a heavy aerial bomb halfway again . . . and again . . . and again . . . until one would land right on top of us.

Artillerymen call the process "walking them in". The method allows them to make recalculations of direction and trajectory until the direct hit is accomplished. To me it was a distorted version of Russian roulette. But somebody else was pulling the trigger.

Other than the fear of getting blown away by the

in-coming rockets and mortars, psychologically the toughest part of the radio relay job, for me, was hearing the chaos of the troops in the field getting blown away. All while I listened on my headset, adjusted the frequencies on the radios, and rearranged circuit cords on the patch panel, trying to keep their communications up and running during their firefights. Sometimes the signals died out and I couldn't help but wonder if the guy on the other end just got killed.

No matter how bad the shit storms were around me, I didn't dare leave my post for fear of someone not getting what they needed if I wasn't doing my job.

****

On quiet nights, I was able to help some grunts and many other guys get through to the satellite station called MARS (Military Affiliate Radio Service). It was the only way for soldiers to call home and talk to their families.

On one of those occasions, I helped a guy who was trying to report unauthorized killings to the press. The signals were weak, but he kept saying he needed to report war crimes to his father who was a newspaper reporter. He claimed his life was at risk from his own people, including his commanders, because they knew he was freaking out about mass murder that had been committed. He claimed the officers involved were trying to cover up crimes.

I never saw his face. I never knew his name. He had a friend that worked one of the radio relay stations out in the field. And his friend had put him through to me by using the order wire, which was only supposed to be used by the operators for maintenance purposes or emergency circumstances. His friend had decided this was an emergency and let him make the call.

I got him through to the satellite station but had no way of following up on whether or not he was able to get through to his father—or whether he survived the ordeal and made it home at the end of his tour. And I never did learn which massacre the guy was trying to report. Sometimes I'm haunted by the shaky, paranoid voice of that soldier trying to report the murders of unarmed Vietnamese civilians including old men, women, and children. I never figured out if he was talking about the massacre at My Lai village or at the village of Thanh Phong—both of which involved the unnecessary killing of civilians. In both tragedies, infantry soldiers claimed they were just following orders from their commanders. Neither massacre reached the news available to the public until after I returned to the United States.

My memory of this experience epitomizes the dilemma I struggle with when I try to accept my responsibility for participating in the war in the first place. But, I am sure I did the right thing when I helped this guy get through to the MARS station.

Some grunts think the support troops are being disloyal to them when we won't tolerate such behavior on the part of the offending members of the infantry by helping to report crimes they commit. The struggle to do the right thing is a heavy burden. I also wonder about my level of responsibility for providing communication if, unbeknownst to me, my job aided in the killing of innocent non-combatants like what happened at both of these villages.

The My Lai village massacre, which happened on March 16, 1968—five days after I entered the Army. I didn't even know the name of the village until an independent investigative journalist reported the incident on November 12, 1969.

The story aired on CBS television and on the Associated Press wire service, while *Time*, *Life*, and *Newsweek* magazines published articles about it. After what I saw and heard in-country, the news didn't surprise me at all. By that time, I had been home for almost a month. When the people around me expressed their shock by the news, they didn't appreciate my response when I said, "What do you think happens in a war zone?"

The Thanh Phong raid occurred on February 25, 1969, during my time in-country. I didn't know the name of that village or hear about the raid until 2001 when the *New York Times* reported the story, three years after the government released the "after-action reports."

Ever since then, I have wondered about how many other incidents occurred during the war that have yet to be made public. But I do know that not all of them were committed by the United States military. The VC and the NVA were just as guilty of war crimes as any Americans, and from what I understand now, even more so.

CHAPTER TEN

I was concerned about my role in exposing possible war crimes, and the likelihood that the commanders may have been trying to cover them up. I couldn't get it out of my mind. I may be unnecessarily paranoid. But retribution was not an uncommon consequence in the environment surrounding me at the time.

Still, life in-country moved along at its usual pace. Each day was different. Some days were calm and uneventful, while other days were filled with red alerts, shit storms, and the general animosity between the infantry soldiers and the support personnel, and the NCOs and the officers. It was during that time that I learned several new lessons about life in the military, especially in a combat zone.

Along one section of our perimeter adjacent to the motor pool, the company mechanics had placed decommissioned and partly destroyed motor vehicles: jeeps, armored personnel carriers, and a variety of trucks. The junk had been there for so long, the jungle vegetation had grown dense around it between the junkyard and our perimeter wire.

The dilapidated vehicles were invisible to the human eye. You couldn't tell it was a vehicular graveyard at all. If you looked at the area from certain angles, you'd swear you were looking at some kind of sculptured topiary mirage of animals and alien beings. And it was even more of a haunting site during the night when you looked at it through the strange lights from the explosions of rockets and mortars, and the illumination flares being dropped from helicopters.

A group of industrious potheads got the bright idea of taking advantage of this oddity. They cut a secret entrance through the undergrowth into the junkyard and used it like a clubhouse. On one of my nights off from my regular duties, I made the mistake of joining them for one of their parties. I crawled through the bramble bush, entering their den.

Beers and joints were being passed around freely. Music was playing but at a low volume for fear of being caught by the upper echelon. However, the atmosphere remained festive: antiwar news, rock and roll music, sports, and girls were the focus of everyone's conversations.

Even though I could hear the usual sounds of small-arms fire and explosions in the background, the sense of freedom was exhilarating. I was off duty and by now, after having been in-country for several months, the noises were almost a comforting backdrop, like the sound effects of a music festival disrupted by the constant whooping noises from helicopter rotor blades. It was like a rock and roll concert in the Nam. Strobe light reflections flickered through the brush from the intermittent illuminations of the night sky being lit up from the popping flares, which were visible throughout the thick jungle canopy above us.

Then suddenly, the sounds of the hovering choppers above our mysterious shelter were joined by the captain's voice on a bull horn yelling, "Get the hell out of there, you idiots. We thought you were a bunch of gooks, and we were ready to blast your asses to kingdom come."

We all panicked and scattered like rabbits through a burrow. I felt like one of those scared little bunnies in the book *Watership Down*. But we all made it back to our bunks without getting caught and at least pretended to be sleeping, for fear of being discovered as part of the motley crew.

In the morning, I couldn't believe my eyes. On my way

to the mess hall for breakfast, the collection of disabled vehicles was in plain sight, clearly visible in the bright daylight. Word passed through the chow line that the captain was so pissed off about the clubhouse in the junkyard that he sprayed the place with Agent Orange as we scattered.

I was surprised by the chemical's immediate killing effect on the vegetation, but I was horrified that our commanders had intentionally sprayed us with Agent Orange. I had never heard of Agent Orange before I was drafted. But during our training, we learned that it's a toxic chemical used by the United States military to kill the jungle vegetation: trees, bushes, plants, and any other life forms that could possibly provide cover for enemy combatants.

It wasn't until nearly 40 years later I found out the hard way that the toxic effects of that deadly defoliant severely damaged my heart.

****

When the level of threat for possible enemy action in our area of operation was low the alert status was considered white. During those periods Army regulations allowed the commissioned officer that was in charge of the signal center where I worked at night to leave a non-commissioned officer in charge. This was common practice in our company. Everybody knew that after all the preparation work at the signal center was completed, the commissioned officer in charge would leave the center and go to the officer's club to have a few drinks with his buddies and watch whatever show was playing that night. In his absence, the non-commissioned officer would be responsible for all of the enlisted men.

However, once the non-commissioned officer was content with the status of things, he would assign one of the enlisted men as the temporary sergeant in charge. We called that person the *acting jack*. A temporary armband with a set of sergeant stripes were pinned on the acting jack's uniform to make it look official. Then the non-commissioned officer would take off and join his friends at his club.

The vast majority of those on duty at night were enlisted men. So, our chances of getting a night at the enlisted men's club were far less than the opportunities available to the higher-ranking members of the night crew. Naturally, resentment towards this unfair practice developed amongst the troops. To offset this inequitable situation, the enlisted men created our own system of allocating extra privileges for ourselves.

It was really very simple. After the bosses were gone, the acting jack gave various orders to the rest of us in his charge. One of us would usually be sent back to the company area to secure an assortment of items for our nightly vigil at the signal center: decks of cards, books to read, and games to play. That made the evenings for the rest of us more enjoyable. A second person was chosen to attend the night's show at the enlisted men's club—the most enviable of positions each night. We saw nothing wrong with this routine. The acting jack was in charge; therefore, the military chain of command was in proper order.

On one of those nights, the acting jack said, "Sully, it's your turn to go to the club."

I didn't waste any time going. I knew a pretty young Vietnamese girl was going to be doing a Janice Joplin impersonation. When I got to the club, I joined a group of my friends at a table in the middle of the crowd.

About halfway through a great performance, we got hit with 122-mm rockets and 80-mm rocket propelled grenades. When the first rounds hit, I knew I couldn't panic because I needed to get back to the signal center. So, instead of diving into the protective bunkers right outside the club, like everybody else, I started running for the signal center. But the shelling was too close and too rapid. Dirt and shrapnel filled the air all around me. The explosions were deafening. I was afraid for my life, but I didn't want to get killed while away from my duty area. My training was ingrained in me by that point. I dropped to the ground and crawled the rest of the way, dragging myself through the dirt and into the signal center.

When I got there, Sergeant DeCoste was standing in front of the patch panel. He looked totally confused, like an octopus with too many tentacles trying to operate the circuit control wires and in-put jacks. As I crawled through the opening, he looked down at me and started screaming.

"Where the fuck were you when this shit storm started? These communication lines need to be kept open."

I jumped up from the floor and said, "Get out of my way."

I took over the patch panel and got things back in order in a very short time. It was quite simple. He had been using the wrong identifying codes. He hadn't been keeping up with the changes being made on a daily basis, which is a routine part of the job for all of us. The shit storm lasted an hour or so, and then everything settled down for the rest of the night.

****

The next morning, the CQ runner came to me at the mess hall during breakfast and told me the captain wanted to see me at 0900. When I walked into the captain's office, Sergeant DeCoste and Lieutenant McKnight, his superior, were already present, standing in the at-ease position. I saluted and stood at attention.

The captain said, "Stand at ease, Private Sullivan. What happened at the signal center last night during that shit storm? I've already heard from these two. Just tell me your side of the story."

"Well, Captain, it was my turn to go to the show after all the prep work was done for the relays and patch-panel work. I was sitting there at the club when the first rocket exploded. I started running for the signal center, but they were blowing up all around me. It was too dangerous for me to be running in an upright position. So, I dropped to the ground and low crawled through the shit storm. When I got to the signal center, Sergeant DeCoste was trying to work the patch panel. But he had all the codes screwed up. So, I took over and straightened them out and got everything back in order."

"Then you admit that you were not at your duty station when Sergeant DeCoste got to the center."

"Yes, Captain."

"You know that could mean you receive an article fifteen for being AWOL."

"That may be true, Captain. But with all due respect, if it comes to that I would prefer a court-martial because I did nothing wrong. I was not away from my duty station without permission. I had permission from the sergeant in charge at the time."

The captain did a quick double take, and followed up my answer with, "DeCoste, you were supposed to be the sergeant in charge last night. Did you give Sullivan permission to go to the show?"

Sergeant DeCoste answered, "No Sir, I did not."

With an angry voice, the captain said, "Who's telling the truth."

I said, "Captain, again with all due respect, I didn't say that Sergeant DeCoste gave me permission. I said the sergeant in charge at the time gave me permission."

"What the hell does that mean?" The captain shouted, with even more anger in his voice.

I proceeded with a comprehensive explanation to the captain about the differences between the protocols and routines that had been going on at the signal center during the night shift for the whole time I had been working there.

I ended with, "None of the enlisted men actually want to be in charge as the acting jack. We don't like having to boss each other around. And if the non-commissioned officers and the commissioned officers can leave the signal center and go to a show at the club, we should be able to as well."

The captain said, "Sergeant DeCoste, is Private Sullivan telling me the truth?"

Sergeant DeCoste began rubbing the back of his neck as he hesitated and then finally answered, "Yes, Captain."

Over the next few days, the captain conducted his own little investigation. Ronnie's parting gesture of good will paid off. All the guys involved backed me up. But the captain called me back into his office at the end of the week and said, "Once again, Private Sullivan, you've avoided disciplinary action. There will be no article fifteen or courts-martial."

He was obviously frustrated.

"Technically you did nothing wrong, but I've got to save face in front of the men and maintain discipline. So, I'm giving you a direct order. For the next two weeks, when you're done at the signal center, you are to spend two hours each morning painting the company shit houses, latrines, and water buffalo right out in plain sight of company formation, where we can all see you. Is there any argument, Private Sullivan?"

"No, Captain."

CHAPTER ELEVEN

When I finished my painting assignments, the captain gave me another special assignment. It was an assignment that brought me so close to the dark side of my soul, I became afraid of what I was capable of doing—especially in a war zone.

He put me in charge of maintaining the M60 machine gun that had been assigned to our company. It was nicknamed "the pig" because the gun's weight and the amount of ammunition it consumed made it difficult for only one soldier to operate. The weapon fired bullets so fast, ammunition needed to be fed into it from belts of 200–1,000 rounds.

Usually a crew of two or three soldiers in an infantry squad would service an M60: the gunner, assistant gunner, and the ammunition bearer. But seeing that we were primarily responsible for keeping radio-relay equipment up and running, no matter what was going on around us, the commanders decided we needed at least one weapon of that magnitude for defensive purposes during shit storms—in case the enemy tried to overrun our area of operation.

But the captain believed there was no chance that our company would be overrun or be sent out on infantry maneuvers. So, he decided that I could handle the job myself. When I complained about not being trained to operate the pig, he got upset and said, "Get the maintenance manual from the quartermaster. Study it. Start taking the gun apart and cleaning it every morning after your night shift is over, learn about the weapon, and be prepared to use it if necessary."

Although I was not a gung-ho infantry soldier when I arrived in Vietnam, I have to admit once I began caring for the M60, it created a certain level of exhilaration in me—a feeling I found disconcerting. After I got over being pissed off about getting more extra duties, I took an interest in the high-powered weapon and accepted the challenge of learning how to operate and maintain the beast.

Feeling the awesome power of the weapon and the destruction it was capable of creating caused an excitement in me that sent me through a kind of spiritual crisis. I wanted a chance to use the thing, a feeling I had never experienced before.

I couldn't understand myself. Such a desire contradicted my personal beliefs, the ones as a practicing Catholic I had been raised to value. I began ignoring the fact that I originally questioned the reasons why I was even fighting in this particular war that I initially didn't believe in, or understand why our government got involved in the first place.

The other side of my new split personality wanted to prove I was a killer, a brave bastard—capable of doing anything and everything anybody else could do, especially the grunts. I changed my mind about jump school and tried to volunteer to go to an infantry outfit, walk point, jump out of planes and helicopters. But before I could reconcile my spiritual crisis, reality caught up with me.

On my next night of guard duty, I was appointed as the CQ runner. I ran errands for the CQ and the sergeant of the guard all night. About 0400 hours, 122-mm rockets and 80-mm rocket propelled grenades came screaming into our company area. Explosions were going off all around me: dirt, shrapnel, and fires breaking out everywhere. Andy, one of my hooch mates, came running up from the bunker line yelling, "They're coming through the wire."

The now-all-to familiar flushing fluid heat of pulsating blood returned and penetrated my entire being. I had never felt this way before. Perhaps this is what an adrenaline rush is, I thought. My fight or flight response went into overdrive. All I could think of was getting a chance to finally kill the enemy. I was uncomfortably surprised at myself.

I ran back to my hooch, grabbed my rifle, helmet, flak jacket, and web belt with extra ammo and headed for the signal center. But the CQ came running out of company headquarters and hollered.

"Sully, get your M60 and guard the ammo bunker. Tell Cheeseman to leave the generators and go with you. Lieutenant McKnight will cover the patch panel until this is over."

I found Cheeseman and told him to come and help me with the pig. I couldn't believe the irony. Rockets and mortars were exploding all around us. The sounds of the explosions were deafening, pressure pushing in on my eardrums like when you gain altitude in an airplane. Sand, gravel, and red-hot metal sprayed the area like a tornado, bouncing off my helmet and burning my flak jacket. I fully expected the ammo bunker to explode at any moment and end the horror. And we were ordered to protect it. What a joke.

Without a word, as we looked at each other with amazement, a silent agreement was reached between me and

Cheeseman. We took up positions on opposite sides of the ammo bunker. Lying in the dirt, we kept our eyes on it despite being hot, tired and scared shitless. We were prepared to shoot any VC who'd be stupid enough to get close to it.

The shit storm lasted a few hours or so. Fortunately, nobody actually penetrated the wire and the ammo bunker didn't get hit. Cheeseman and I put our gear away and went to the mess hall for breakfast. We sat by ourselves over in a corner, but we couldn't eat anything. We had no appetite and quietly admitted to each other that last night's experience scared the hell out of us more than we had ever imagined.

Although maintaining the M60 brought with it a strange sense of exhilaration, the experience of guarding the ammo bunker reached deep into my soul and made me feel a level of anger I had never experienced. I couldn't tell if I was angry with myself or someone—or something—else.

Like the ancient mystics tell us, when you reach that point, you feel a loss of ego and dying seems to be a better option than living. I questioned whether or not I could live through another shit storm, waiting for the grim reaper to appear and take me away. Rest in peace now had a whole new meaning to me. And it was scary.

Deep down in the depths of my subconscious, I came to

a strange conclusion. Waiting to die seemed to be worse than actually being dead. A spark had ignited a flame that burnt a hole through my heart, and I've wanted to kill anybody that I perceived as a threat to me ever since. It shocked me to feel that way. I felt such an internal conflict that I became afraid of what I might do if another attack should come that close to me again.

****

I knew that before my tour was over, I would have to confront my internal conflicts again and again. By now, my time in Vietnam had proven to me that the old adage, "War is long periods of boredom punctuated by moments of sheer terror," was certainly true and described my experience accurately.

I'm ashamed to admit that for a while, I even contemplated doing something stupid, like one of the guys in our hooch that shot himself in the foot just to get out of the war and be sent home. When they questioned him, he claimed it was an accident while he was cleaning his weapon. He was shipped out and we never found out what happened to him.

For the rest of my tour, when enemy action was slow, I cherished those long periods of boredom. But the usual sounds of small-arms fire at night and the shelling of the mountains provided enough of a background to remind me that I was still in a combat zone. The feeling of comfort it gave me, in such a hostile environment, became an odd sensation that I've never been able to reconcile. Perhaps it was a primal need for peace as a survival technique in the midst of so much ugliness and chaos.

Most of my memories of Vietnam come and go with no real sense of chronological sequence, but the events that took place around holidays, birthdays and special events are easy to place in time. By Thanksgiving, everyone I knew was looking forward to the home-style meal promised to us by our battalion commander.

The meal was delicious and looked so good it made me homesick: glistening golden brown turkey, delicious gravy that felt like velvet as it descended my throat, stimulating taste buds that hadn't been activated since I arrived in-country. Guys I didn't even know knitted themselves right into the seats next to me, amongst other friends that I had known for months by then. Conversation was about our lives back home: family, jobs, girlfriends, best friends, and going back to school. The grunts that were lucky enough to be in for a stand down joined us for the meal without any problems.

We told our favorite jokes; everyone laughed even if they had already heard it before. War stories were frowned upon; nobody wanted to think about that kind of bullshit on a holiday, not even the grunts. But great high school stories of athletic achievements were encouraged. Some guys got choked up as they spoke about home. But another guy would jump right in with a funny comment to keep the atmosphere light. No big theatrical productions of tragedy were allowed at the tables, just companionship and reinforcement. Taking time to rejoice and be appreciative and focusing on gratitude for this moment we were able to enjoy. When the meal was over, we picked up our trays, returned them to the kitchen, grabbed our weapons and went back to our duty stations.

On my way to the signal center, I stopped at the MARS station and was able to call home. I had a quick conversation with my mom and dad, and I could hear the voices of the rest of the family in the background wishing me well, but I didn't have time to talk to anyone else. I assured my parents that I was doing great.

That telephone call left me with mixed emotions. Communicating with family while in a combat zone was difficult. It reminded me how much I missed the love of my family, and the comfort and safety of home. The voices of my parents and the distant voices of my brother and sisters remained a distraction for several days, and I had to push them out of my mind to focus on my responsibilities—especially when dealing with the enemy.

After a few relatively quiet nights of guard duty, I was caught by surprise when my spiritual conflict surfaced once again. On this memorable night, we were on red alert—the highest level of threat of enemy activity. Basically, it was a free-fire zone—kill anything that moved out in the dark. Nobody could sleep in a bunker on those nights.

In the middle of the night I heard strange noises coming from the underbrush outside of the wire. The hair on the back of my neck stood up straight and began to itch. It was driving me crazy. I was scratching like a dog with fleas. The other guys in the bunker, a couple of grunts, told me to settle down. They said, "Don't be such a REMF; you're making us nervous."

It was a dark, moonless night; a little breeze was ruffling the marsh grass between the riverbed and the perimeter wire. You could hear the screechy noises of animals caught in the wire, breathing their last breath. On the other side of the waterline along the banks of the marsh, up in the grass, I could see the flickering of a flame. The shadows around it created a ghostly image of someone carrying a lantern, like they were looking for something they had lost.

Whoever it was, friend or foe, I couldn't tell. They were in an area that was probably a rice paddy, where the friendly villagers were allowed to do their farming during the daylight hours. But at night they were supposed to stay further back, on the other side of the estuary, in their tiny village huts. And they were definitely not allowed to cross the inlet from the sea.

I watched carefully for at least an hour. The light kept moving slowly, closer and closer to where the marshy inlet between the two banks of the small river separated our side from their side. I told the grunts about it. But the shadow person carrying the lantern was hard to see.

After a while he appeared to be lowering himself into one of the woven-reed-basket boats that I watched the villagers fishing in along the shores of the beach on a regular basis during daylight hours. For a short time, I thought it might be just my imagination.

In angry, whispered undertones, the grunts said, "We don't see him. But if you do, take the shot before he shoots us."

I finally caught a clear view and could see him cross to our side and start to climb out of his little craft. He was about a hundred yards away. Before he could start moving toward our bunker, I fought the panic, took a shot at the light, which I could barely see, and the light went out. Immediately, we all heard the splash of something or someone falling into the water.

When the grunts heard the splash, they both screamed, "Next time, don't wait so long. Just shoot the bastard, talk later."

The field phone rang a moment later. One of the grunts answered and said, "We shot a gook carrying a light and coming up out of the marsh, towards our bunker."

The guy at the other end of the radio said, "No sweat. Morning patrol will pick up the body at sunrise."

Nothing else happened the rest of the night. And nobody questioned me about the incident. There was no protocol to counsel a soldier who just killed a man. But it's bothered me ever since. I still wonder whether or not I shot a flickering light or shot the person carrying it.

A Long Triage

CHAPTER TWELVE

After Thanksgiving had come and gone, we were all looking forward to *The Bob Hope Christmas Special*. Since I worked nights and had most days to myself, I went down to the Chu Lai amphitheater bright and early in the morning on the day of the show. But one special forces guy had gotten there before me. That would have been fine, except he had already spread rain ponchos over all the seats of the first three rows to save seats for his friends.

When I saw that I got so pissed off, I headed down to confront him, but one of the guys on the stage doing preparation work for the show jumped down off the stage and came running towards me. He stopped me cold in my tracks.

"I know, man. But before you say anything, I just want

to warn you about that dude."

"What's going on? He can't do that," I said back to him.

He responded, "I know what you mean. But he's one of those LRRPs. We all know those guys are crazy."

"Yeah, I know what they say about them."

"Well, he told me he just survived a major firefight out in the boonies and will kill anyone who tries to stop him from saving seats for him and his pals. The look on his face convinced me that he was serious. So, I left him alone."

I realized this was one of those moments when it's better to hold your tongue. I went over to the guy and asked him if he needed any help because the wind was starting to pick up and the ponchos would start blowing all over if he didn't weight them down.

"Don't fuck with me," he said.

"I'm not. I just wanted to help. I know what you guys have to do out there in the bush. Not that it's great here either."

"Okay, then. What's your idea?"

"Wait a minute."

I ran down to the beach and scrounged up a bunch of buckets: filled them with sand, brought them back, and spread the sand across the ponchos."

"When the wind comes up, the ponchos might flap around a bit, but they won't blow away. You guys can shake off the sand before you sit down for the show."

When his friends arrived, he told them what I had done to help save their seats. Instead of harassing me for being a REMF, they asked me to sit with them, which I did. And we got along fine.

It was really a great show. Ann Margret was the main attraction and Bob Hope was hilarious. The LRRPs were all friendly to me, but I believe they would have given me a hard time if I had just taken one of the front row seats on my own and sat there in the middle of them.

****

The New Year holiday came without much celebration. Some of the hooches including mine still had makeshift Christmas trees standing. A nice meal was available at the mess hall. But rumors had circulated among most of us who were not in-country the year before during the 1968 TET offensive that the enemy was planning another major offensive for the up-coming Vietnamese New Year. The word was that the Tet offensive for 1969 would make the 1968 Tet offensive, a truly devastating event for the US a year ago, look like "child's play."

Military intelligence had us on notice that the offensive would begin sometime between our January New Year holiday and Tet, the Vietnamese New Year. This is celebrated sometime between January 21st and February 20th, based on which animal was to be celebrated for the upcoming calendar year. In 1969, the date was January 28th, the year of the rooster.

We were told that when the Tet offensive arrived, it would be the largest military offensive our enemies would launch during the entire war to date. Once again, I was afraid for my life. But at least I was not a cherry anymore, and I had some idea of what to expect.

I was restless and short-tempered waiting for the big event. To make matters worse, racial tensions between black, white, and Hispanic soldiers had recently escalated to the point that we were ordered to have our M16s locked and loaded and always in our possession until further orders. Tension between grunts and REMFs had escalated as well. We were advised that in addition to a pending threat from the enemy, we needed to defend ourselves from our brothers in arms if necessary.

At first, I found such a concern to be unbelievable. But in the middle of the day, on one of the days I was hanging around the company area with some of my friends instead of going to the beach, I learned another big lesson about being in the military.

One of the grunts, that was in for a stand down, was high as a kite on some mysterious drug that he bought in the village, came running through the area spraying bullets from his M16 like a wild man and screaming.

"I'm going to kill as many of you fucking REMFs as I can."

He was spraying bullets across our hooches, with his weapon set on fully automatic. Besides the ping of the bullets on our metal lockers and the rat-tat-tat of the gun itself, we could see some of our doors splintering as they were hit. When he went to change clips so he could keep firing, a group of us tackled him, brought him to the ground, and called for the MPs to come get him.

Fortunately, no one was hit by any of the bullets. But he scared the shit out of all of us. He put up quite a struggle with the MPs, but they got him restrained and hauled him away. We never saw the guy again or found out what happened to him.

A few nights later, I was the CQ runner making my

rounds through the company area, I witnessed a "friendly-fire" attack on a non-commissioned officer. As I walked by the cable team's hooch, a spark flared up in the corner where I knew the team's sergeant had his bunk. I saw a couple of guys run out the back door just as flames lit up the area around his bunk.

I ran into the hooch grabbed the sleeping drunk sergeant and dragged him out into the company street. I smothered the flames threatening to engulf him by rolling him around in the dirt. I called out to the CQ and he called for the medics. The burnt sergeant and I were both taken to the hospital and checked out by the medical staff. He was alive. They patched him up and kept him in the hospital, and eventually they shipped him out to a different unit. I was okay and released before nightfall that night. And I remained stationed with my company for the remainder of my tour of duty.

The incident was written up as an accident and nothing more was said about it. I knew it was no accident, but I couldn't do anything about it. No one wanted to listen to what I had to say about what really happened that night. So, life went on with no more mention of the incident. But for me, it's just another one of those events that continues to creep into my recurring nightmares.

During our wait for the Vietnamese New Year and the expectation of another Tet offensive, I was placed under orders to keep the M-60 handy at all times, as well as cleaned and operable. And of course, in the event of a shit storm to guard the ammo bunker. But the storm never arrived. Some of the guys expressed disappointment, but not me. By that time, I had lost my interest in the adrenaline rush of combat.

****

In between the holiday season and Saint Patrick's Day, I had another close call. The senior man in each hooch was responsible for supervising and paying the hooch maid. In our hooch, Jared was the senior man during my first seven months in-country. Jared and Lee Lee, our hooch maid, had fallen in love, or so he said but that's another story. He didn't have a girlfriend back home and was quite smitten with Lee Lee.

Jared and Lee Lee planned on getting married. But he had to go back to the states for his discharge from the Army, return to Vietnam, and then marry. Once they were husband and wife, she would be able to return to the states as his wife under a special program that would allow her to become a U.S. citizen.

Lee Lee's family was very excited about the wedding. They invited Jared to bring a few friends to the family home in the Village to celebrate the upcoming event. At that time, Jared, Jack, and I were kind of our own little group. And Jack was going to be Jared's best man. So, the three of us got day passes to leave the base and go to the Village.

We were authorized the use of a duz'n half from the motor pool, but we had to take some grunts with us who also had passes. As we left through the main gate, the MP on duty cautioned us.

"You guys need to be careful, there are reports of VC in the Ville. So, you better stay away."

One of the grunts responded, "We can take care of ourselves."

Jared said, "It's not a problem for us. We're not going to spend time in the Ville. We're going to my fiancé's house, just outside the Village."

"Good luck. You've been warned," said the MP and he let us through the gate.

When we got to the village, the grunts jumped out at one of the local whorehouses.

"Just pick us up here when you're all done with your big wedding party. If we're not outside, just blow the horn and we'll wrap up what we're doing and be right out."

We left the grunts in the village and headed to Lee

Lee's house. It was located near the banks of the Thu Bon River on the edge of the rice paddies. Her family had been farming the land for many generations. It was a typical Vietnamese, earthen-walled, whitewashed, four-cornered, grass-roofed structure with no windows. There was a main door in the front of the house and a door on one side facing a patio surrounded by rows of small stones.

Inside, the home was divided into two areas separated by bamboo curtain walls. One area was for sleeping and the other was sort of a great room used for cooking, eating, and entertaining. We sat in the great room on bamboo mats covering the compacted earthen floor. Just outside, I could see that flat stones made up the floor of the patio. It was covered in whitewash and kept clean for drying rice in the sun. Beyond the rows of stone walls, rice paddies surrounded the curtilage of the family's home.

Lee Lee introduced us to her family and began serving a traditional egg and rice meal. I was quite surprised to find out that eggshells had been ground up and sprinkled throughout the dish. Lee Lee explained this to me after noticing the look of surprise on my face.

Before we even finished eating, the sounds of small-arms fire broke out behind the house and interrupted the meal. The shots kept getting closer and closer to the house. Jared, Jack, and I looked at each other with concern and grabbed our weapons.

The firefight was breaking out between a group of South Vietnamese uniformed soldiers and some of the VC who were in the area.

Lee Lee's parents jumped up, grabbed us by our shirt sleeves, and in their broken English/Vietnamese said, "No GI, no, no, no GI in house. Beaucoup number ten. VC no like—go, go, go now. No VC see GI here."

Jared said, "Let's go. It doesn't matter who wins that battle out there. Either way, her family will be safer if they don't find Americans in the house."

Nobody was going to argue the point, but it bothered us. It was like we were running away from the fight. But we went out the front door anyway. As Jared jumped up into the cab of the truck and got behind the wheel, he said, "Give it a little push. We'll roll down the hill before I start her up, so the VC won't hear us leaving."

Jack and I got behind the truck and gave it a push. Fortunately, it rolled easily down a slight grade. And when we were a safe distance from the house, Jared started the truck. We stopped at the whorehouse for the grunts, but nobody was out front.

Jared said, "I'm not blowing any horn. The VC back

there will hear it. Jack, run in and get those guys. Sully, guard the back of the truck."

When I went around to the back of the truck, a crowd of Vietnamese kids had gathered around to see what all the excitement was about. I saw a grenade rolling out of the crowd and through the dirt headed towards the back wheels of our truck.

I could see the pin had already been pulled. But an elastic band was wrapped around the pineapple body holding the handle tight in place. So, I knew it was safe, at least for the moment.

As I reached down and grabbed the grenade, I noticed a little Vietnamese girl, probably about twelve years old, running away from the crowd. I took aim. The crowd parted like Moses and the Red Sea. But I wasn't even sure she was the culprit who was trying to blow up the truck. And I hesitated from shooting a little kid. I just couldn't do it.

Just as I was taking aim, Jack and the grunts were coming out of the whorehouse. When they saw me holding the grenade and watching the girl run away, they could tell I wasn't going to shoot the her. One of the grunts said, "You REMFs are all the same. You should've taken the shot."

I said, "The hell with you," and tossed the grenade

to him and followed up with, "Here man, put a pin in this." But I kept my weapon locked and loaded, with my finger on the trigger staring at him. And the whole way back into the base I didn't take my eyes off the grunts. One of them fumbled around in his gear and found something to use as a pin for the grenade and inserted it into the empty hole to disarm the explosive device.

Nobody said anything else the whole way back to the base. Jared pulled the truck up to the grunts stand-down area. They jumped down from the truck, remained quiet, and disappeared into the crowd.

Jared, Jack, and I returned the truck to the motor pool. They both said, "Sully, it don't mean nothing." And nobody ever mentioned that day again.

CHAPTER THIRTEEN

When Jared completed all his arrangements to marry Lee Lee, our hooch needed to hire a new hooch maid. By then, I was the senior man in hooch number five. And my first responsibility was to hire the new maid. Lee Lee brought her younger sister Tran onto the base to train her for the job. And I went ahead and said it was fine with me. That's where the problem started.

Unbeknownst to me, one of the cafeteria workers had claimed the job to be hers. Evidently the Vietnamese had some kind of seniority system of their own. The hooch maids earned more money than the cafeteria workers, especially when the maids got tips for performing extra work. So, the veteran cafeteria workers expected to be promoted to hooch maids when the opportunities became available.

At suppertime on that first night when Lee Lee's sister had come onto the base to be trained for the job, the woman who was claiming the job to be hers threatened me as I was going through the chow line. She spoke with a great deal of anger in her voice with a variety of broken English mixed with Vietnamese

"Number one GI give Tran new job."

I tried my best to explain to her that Lee Lee and Jared had arranged for Lee Lee's sister to take over Lee Lee's hooch-maid job.

Her face turned red and she screamed.

"No give Tran job. You, number ten GI. . . You die tonight!"

I reported the cafeteria worker's threat to our company commander. He said there was nothing he could do unless we were hit that night. Sure enough, in the middle of that night, several 80-mm rockets exploded right next to my hooch spraying shrapnel and gravel all around. Nobody was injured, but it scared the hell out of us.

The captain had the woman's base privileges revoked. We never saw her again. And Lee Lee's little sister remained our hooch-maid for the rest of my time in-country.

****

Towards the end of March, on my way to the signal center to start my night shift, I was carrying a load of stuff for the night's entertainment and thinking about calling my family again by the satellite phone at the MARS station to wish my twin sisters a happy birthday. But that thought was interrupted by the screech of sirens piercing my ears. That sound always penetrated my eardrums and scared me half to death.

I started running towards the signal bunker. But rocket-propelled grenades and 122-mm rockets started exploding all around me. I ran faster and faster. My only thought was to get to my duty station. Time seemed to slow down as the explosions got closer and closer.

As I was running, I could hear the fluttering propeller of a rocket propelled grenade in my right ear. It was like the thing was following me. As I approached the opening in the ground that led into the signal bunker, I saw Cheeseman operating the generators on the hill above me. I screamed as loud as I could. "Cheeseman, they're coming in right behind me."

He screamed back, "Hit the dirt. I'm coming right on top of you."

As I dove towards the black hole, Cheeseman slammed into me in midair. Together we flew piggyback style towards the canvas flap covering the entryway. As we landed on the ground with him on top of me, out of the corner of my eye I saw the brightest flash of light I've ever seen and heard an explosion that blew out my eardrums.

The stuff I was carrying splattered all over the ground and went every which way: magazines, playing cards, sodas, and sandwiches. I turned my head and spit the dirt out of my mouth. When I did, I couldn't believe my eyes. Cheeseman's hair was standing straight up like the needles on a prickly porcupine and it was albino white, instead of its usual reddish blonde. His eyes were wide open with the hollow blank stare of a dead man looking out into the great abyss.

The guys in the bunker pulled him of me and told me to get to the patch panel and get the communications back online. They called the medics to come and get Cheeseman. I never saw him again or heard any news about how he made out after he was evacuated.

I was devasted when I relived this incident years later during my post-surgery delirium.

****

About a week later, I had to go out with the cable team

one night to help troubleshoot some of our faulty circuit connections. Just like back home, the cables and wires connected communication centers: radio relays, telephone terminals, and the end users. And cables and wires ran from antennas and telephone poles rising into the sky.

Unfortunately for those of us responsible for keeping the lines of communication open, our presence while maintaining the outdoor equipment made us exposed to the enemy and vulnerable to attack, and the VC knew exactly where all the communication equipment was located. The landlines ran out of the back end of the bunker and up a series of telephone poles.

The first group of poles surrounded the bunker, and the wires extended out in all directions across a network of telephone poles in series, simple, parallel and combination circuitry terminating at the various command posts like a spider web. The resulting web provided contact between everyone depending on radio, telephone, telegraph, and teletype communications.

Although nobody got shot that night, I still have nightmares of the experience, just the same. I think it's because we had been extremely vulnerable out in the dark, climbing those poles and checking the wires and not knowing if snipers were watching our every move.

****

Living through shit storms of rockets and mortars falling out of the sky, listening to the rat-tat-tat of small arms fire, and the enemy trying to penetrate the perimeter became so commonplace that when the environment was quiet and peaceful, it seemed strange. During the quiet times, as long as I did my job at the signal center and shared guard duty without complaining, my commanding officer left me alone.

I had been lucky enough to buy a surfboard for twenty-five dollars from an Australian soldier who was going home and couldn't bring it with him. Unless I was on duty at the signal center or pulling guard duty, I was able to spend my time down at the beach in my own little semi-private world. Other guys would show up and borrow my stuff, smoke pot, drink beer, and generally just hang out hiding from their superiors. Some of them were grunts in for a stand down or what they called in-country rest and relaxation.

A few times I had to deal with the REMF versus grunt bullshit. But when that derogatory attitude reared its ugly head on the beach, I simply challenged the grunts to spend a night with me in the signal center. Most of them said no thanks.

But the guys who did accept my challenge never made it through a whole night. When they heard the eerie sounds of the enemy walking explosive rounds of rockets and mortars towards our location from someplace above and beyond the bunker the grunts would say, "Okay, man, I see what you mean. We're like sitting ducks in here with nowhere to go. At least out in the bush we can move around, defend ourselves, and try to get away from this kind of shit."

Then they would leave and never harass me again. But they must have told their friends about the surfboard I had available at the beach because more of them kept showing up to borrow it from me during their stand-downs. And eventually the harassment evaporated.

Around the end of May, two grunts showed up at the beach with a duffel bag full of pot, a tent, and a cot to sleep in. They set up their camp under a row of trees along a shaded section of the beach, which was hard to see unless you knew it was there. They came to me and borrowed my surfboard for several days. We got along pretty well considering they were grunts and I was "just a REMF".

They shared their pot generously and sat around telling war stories that were hard to believe or respect. Of course, I only listened and kept my mouth shut until they left, it wasn't worth getting into it with them. What I wanted to tell them was that they were either exaggerating or they were sick in the head. They bragged about their kills, even the ones they made while not engaged in combat with the enemy.

One of the guys from an engineering company's road crew thought it was funny that he ran over an old Vietnamese man who didn't run fast enough to get out of the way of the road grader he was driving. Another guy said he felt bad about the old man he shot for beating a dog. But he said he saved the dog and kept it as the company pet.

These guys weren't the only ones who enjoyed bragging about their violent behavior. I heard so many stories that I wasn't sure which ones to believe or not. The one I did believe was a guy who said he had eighty confirmed kills while walking point for seven months. He was being sent home on a section eight psychological discharge. He shot a nun carrying a school bag over her shoulder. He believed she was responsible for setting the booby traps that had killed several of his friends.

After he shot her, he got into a fight with the young lieutenant in charge of the patrol and hadn't been in-country very long. The lieutenant freaked out, believing the nun was a civilian casualty. He threatened to court-martial the soldier and a fistfight broke out between the two.

But when the medics with the patrol went to give aid to the woman, they opened up the school bag she was carrying and found that it was full of explosive devices. Obviously, everyone present knew the guy was justified in shooting her, but he was being shipped out anyway.

I believed his story because of what I saw in his eyes, heard in his voice, and felt in his presentation when telling the story. He was somewhere in outer space mentally. It was scary just to be around him. I could tell that he was a dangerous character, someone not to fool around with.

A Long Triage

CHAPTER FOURTEEN

For me Memorial Day marks the beginning of summer. Back home, it usually means the end of cool weather and the beginning of many beach days ahead. My hometown is a coastal village where Memorial Day is second only to the 4th of July in terms of how we celebrate. And summer extends all the way to Labor Day, the first Monday in September.

After Memorial Day weekend is over, I had always looked forward to my birthday on June 10th. But now it comes with a certain trepidation. On June 8, 1969, just two days shy of my 21st birthday, when my night shift was over as usual at 0600, I crawled out of the bunker and entered into a beautiful, sunny day. It was days like this that I felt blessed to have the night shift so I could enjoy the sunshine. As a lifelong beach lover, this was a salvation of sorts in an otherwise fucked up place. I skipped breakfast at the mess hall and went down to the beach.

There was a slight offshore breeze and the waves were about as good as they got during the summer in Chu Lai. I picked up my surfboard from my tent and ran down to the water's edge, jumped in, and paddled out. I was the only one at the beach.

I caught a nice wave and almost forgot where I was. In my mind, I had entered that mystical world where surfers feel like they're in God's hands, where the beautiful hue of the sea becomes one with the greenish glow and frothing white of breaking waves. Suddenly, a loud swooshing noise passed by me. The sea erupted all around me in a fountain of ocean spray and knocked me off my board.

When I surfaced and caught my breath, I could hear the screeching sounds of alarms and hear the explosions of rockets and mortars. I looked up and could see the shit storm was covering the entire beach and working its way towards the hospital on the cliff above me. The next round exploded on the medevac helipad right next to the hospital. Then the hospital was hit. I was scared out of my mind.

Even now when I think back on that day, I find it hard to believe that I took the time to grab my board, put it back in my tent, low crawl through the exploding rockets and mortars, and make it to the signal center. When I got there, I jumped in and helped out the guys on duty until the shit storm ended. I was told to go back to my bunk, get some sleep, and come back at 1800 for my regular night shift.

The next morning when the day crew came to relieve me, they told me that a rocket hit the hospital and when it exploded, some of the shrapnel flew through the air, hit one of the Army nurses, slit her throat, and killed her instantly. I was horrified when I heard that news. I knew I had seen the explosion that killed her, and I had survived through the same shit storm while I was surfing and crawling across the beach to get to the signal center.

The guilt was overwhelming. But what could I have done? I had performed my duties under enemy fire as I had been trained to do. She was going to be killed no matter what I did. As it turns out, she was the only American woman killed in Vietnam by hostile enemy fire. It may have hit me extra hard because my mother served in Europe during WWII as an Army nurse, and she had served under enemy fire.

The next day was my birthday. I stayed at the beach by myself and didn't celebrate. I kept thinking about the shit storm and the death of the nurse while I surfed. Nobody bothered me. My friends knew I wanted to be left alone. And the captain gave me the night off for my birthday, and I had no daytime duties. Even now, I can't help but think of her when I go to the beach. Survivor's guilt is a strange thing to feel. It's strong and powerful and relentless. I wonder if it ever goes away.

****

A few days after the Fourth of July, the captain assigned me to help set up the communication equipment for the relay operations at a new firebase that was being established out in the boonies. It was about a hundred miles from my company area. It was so new it didn't have a name yet. I packed up all my personal gear and reported to the helipad for my ride out to the landing zone.

I waited for thirty-six hours without sleep before the chopper finally came to get me. I started to climb aboard. But before I could hop in, I was stopped by the crew chief. He said, "Never mind. Those poor suckers got overrun and we lost the hill. You can get some rest and go back to your regular duties."

I was horrified. Guilt set in again, like the shit storm that killed the nurse, I had missed another close call. The chopper that had come to pick me up was on its third trip out to the firebase when it was called back. It had been late coming in to get me because it was giving support to the guys on the ground during the firefight. If it hadn't been overloaded on its second trip, I would have already been at the LZ and dead with the rest of the replacement troops.

****

In August, I finally got my chance to go on leave for rest and relaxation, my first time out of Vietnam in almost a year. I chose to go to Australia. When I got there, I decided not to spend my time and money drinking and carousing around the Kings Cross section of Sydney, where most of the guys on R&R were going. That's where the barrooms and hookers were located. I had had enough of that kind of low-life atmosphere during the few times I took trips to the villages of Anh Ton and Nha Trang in Vietnam.

I wanted to meet real Australians, regular ordinary people, and experience as much normalcy as I could find. So, I joined up with a couple guys I had met on the plane who felt the same way I did. We shared a taxicab and got away from the airport. The cab driver asked us for an address, but we couldn't give him one. We told him about our intentions to avoid the chaos and confusion at Kings Cross, and he said he knew exactly where to take us.

He dropped us off at a traffic circle just outside the main entrance to the University of New South Wales, Kensington, Australia. The campus, filled with pretty girls, was right across the street from where we got out of the cab.

It was August, the end of their winter season. The temperature was hovering around sixty degrees Fahrenheit, which is pretty warm to me, being from New England. And it was great to get out of Vietnam for part of the rainy season. A car full of girls drove by in a convertible with the top down. We waved to them. The car turned around and came back to where we were standing on the traffic circle.

The girls were laughing a lot and we asked them, "What's so funny." The three of them mockingly chanted together, "You guys must be lost. Kings Cross is on the other side of town."

The three of us chimed back, "We're not looking for Kings Cross."

One of the girls said, "Why not? That's where all you American boys go for cheap thrills."

"We're not like everybody else. We don't need cheap thrills. We'd rather meet the real Australians."

They were all pretty good looking and must have had a soft spot for American soldiers trying to avoid the mayhem of Kings Cross. Two of them had the stereotypical blonde hair we expected of Australian women; the one who looked to be the oldest, was adorned with flaming red hair with a sheen that reflected the sunlight with a glow.

"Well then, mates. We'll take you home to meet the family. We're all Millers," said the redhead.

As it turned out, they were sisters. We met their mom, dad, and their brother who was a cop. We spent all week with them: had meals at their home most days, went swimming at Bondi Beach with them, ate at family restaurants, and went to the movies twice. We even watched the Woodstock Music Festival on the family's television set.

During the show, they kept asking, "Are all you Americans that crazy."

We just laughed it off saying, "Not us."

It was a great week. We exchanged addresses and promised to write to each other. When we left, all three of us felt a little bit more normal until we reported back to Vietnam. Unfortunately, I was the only one of the three of us to make it out of Vietnam alive. The other two guys were killed in separate firefights within a week after returning to their units.

The Millers and I wrote to each other during the remainder of my tour and for several years after I returned home. In their letters to me, they reiterated an open invitation for me to come back to Australia and visit them.

A Long Triage

****

When I returned to Vietnam after my week in Australia, I decided to apply for re-admittance to college and finish my education when I got home. In addition to the application, transcripts, and letters of recommendations, I was required to pass a physical exam before I could be accepted for the second semester starting in January 1970.

The letters of recommendation and transcripts were not difficult to obtain. But getting the physical examination while in Vietnam turned out to be an emotionally difficult experience for me. The deadline for applying required me to submit my full application package to the admissions office by September 30, 1969, and I wouldn't be home until October 14, 1969.

In order to obtain the physical examination, I had to get in line with the walking-wounded and local civilians at the evacuation hospital and hope that a doctor would find the time to help me out. Considering the conditions of the people surrounding me, part of me could only feel spoiled and selfish.

While waiting my turn for the doctor, I sat alongside a little Vietnamese girl. She had several open bullet holes in her arms and legs. But the amazing thing that sticks in my mind was how happy she and her mother appeared to be because they appreciated the care the girl was receiving from the American doctors.

Their attitude certainly put things into perspective for me. The long wait for my physical didn't matter anymore. I contemplated the enormity of this war and its civilian casualties. For the thousandth time, I asked myself why we were fighting this war; I could never find an answer. All these years later, I can still see a picture of that little girl in my mind as though I just met her yesterday.

****

OCTOBER 1969:

When it got close to my time to leave Vietnam, I had no more guard duties or special details to perform in my company area. My replacement at the signal center was scheduled to take over my duties on the tenth of October, and I had orders to report back to the same reception center I arrived at when I first landed in Chu Lai at the opposite end of the base.

When I got there, I thought it hadn't changed much. But at least this time I didn't see any rats in the trenches around the area. While we waited for our flight orders, as enlisted men, we were expected to perform some of the housekeeping duties. At least the sergeant in charge didn't send us out to the bunker line. But we did have to wash pots and pans, peel potatoes, and burn shit.

Of course, as a short-timer, I believed I shouldn't have had to do anything. So, I had a bad attitude. To make matters worse, the personnel clerk couldn't find my orders. I had already been in-country for twenty-two extra days, and the clerk said it would take him at least three more to get me on a flight to Cam Rahn Bay. From there, the planes we all called *freedom birds* took off on a daily basis for home.

I was really annoyed and said, "I'll get my own ride."

"Good luck," the clerk responded. "The last guy who tried that went home in a body bag."

"You don't scare me with bullshit like that. I'll be out of here before you straighten out your stupid paperwork, and you can give my spot to some other lucky bastard."

I went over to the helipad next to my company area and hooked a ride on a chopper. I knew what I was doing because I had done the same thing when I went to Nha Trang and Australia for R&R.

The pilot said he would take me along but warned me that he was on standby and could be called in for a mission at any time. I knew that meant I would be expected to help out if he was called in for a medevac or to support an infantry outfit. But I was willing to take that chance. He also said he couldn't guarantee he would get me all the way to Cam Rahn Bay, but at least he would get me closer to where I was going. I gladly accepted all of those conditions. I just wanted to get out of Vietnam.

I climbed aboard and we headed south. We didn't get too far before he got called into an LZ to pick up a small group of Republic of Korea Marines from the White Horse Brigade. Four of them had been in a bunker outside the airbase at Pleiku in the Central Highlands.

A 122-mm rocket had hit them. One was already dead, but the other three were still breathing. When we got there, the medics had the wounded patched up pretty good. I helped carry them on stretchers to the chopper, and then we flew to the airbase. When we arrived, the medics still needed my help with the stretchers. We got the wounded off the chopper and loaded them into an Air Force hospital plane.

I was about ready to get off the plane when the pilot called out, "Hold up there! My crew tells me you're a short-timer looking for a ride to Cam Rahn Bay. Thanks for your help! We're headed for Cam Rahn now with these poor guys. You're welcome to come along and help us out again, and then report for your flight home."

I happily replied, "Sure, Captain, thanks a lot." I felt relieved. I had taken a chance that had paid off, and I wasn't still sitting back in Chu Lai waiting for the clerks to straighten out their paperwork.

The flight to Cam Rahn Bay went smoothly. We landed without incident. I helped the medics get the stretchers into the hospital. After the orderlies in the emergency room took the patients, I ran outside and caught a ride from a guy driving a jeep. He took me over to the airstrip. I showed my orders to the clerks at the airbase and begged my way onto the next flight home.

Welcome to My War

ACKNOWLEDGEMENTS

The author would like to thank the people listed below for their valuable help in completing this work of Creative Non-fiction.

Carol Saint John
Green Valley, Arizona

Christopher Anderson
Eastern Point Lit house
Gloucester, Massachusetts

Damaris Herlihy
Curran Press
Charlotte, Vermont

Laurie Fielding
Gloucester, Massachusetts

Dorothy Nelson
Veterans Writing Workshop
Gloucester, Massachusetts

ABOUT THE AUTHOR

Francis J. Sullivan Jr. Was born on June 10, 1948 in Cambridge Massachusetts. He moved with his family to Rockport Massachusetts after several years of spending vacations in the seaside community located north of Boston on Cape Ann.

Graduating from Rockport High School in 1966, he then attended college for his freshman year and was drafted into the US Army in March of 1968. Mr. Sullivan served in Vietnam from September of 1968 to October of 1969.

Upon returning from Vietnam Mr. Sullivan attempted to complete his college education at Salem State College in Salem Massachusetts. As a result of the tumultuous atmosphere across America during the protesting of the 1960's and 1970's he became disenchanted with his native country and immigrated to Australia.

His experience in Australia led him to conclude that America was no worse than other nations across the globe, and he returned home to complete his undergraduate work, teach school for twenty years, marry, raise a family and graduate from law school.

Like many of his fellow Vietnam veterans, he has struggled with the invisible wounds of war including, Agent Orange related heart disease, PTSD, and tinnitus. On January 14, 2014 he experienced a Spontaneous Subdural Hematoma and underwent a craniotomy to evacuate the pooling blood. He believes this injury is also a consequence of his war time experiences.

He has written A Long Triage in an effort to heal himself and believes that readers will find universal themes throughout his story, which apply to society in general. He also believes that making his story public will contribute to his healing process.

Mr. Sullivan hopes his story will also contribute to a better understanding of what the long-term effects of war have on not only the soldiers who have visible physical injuries but also those who suffer with injuries that cannot be seen by the naked eye.